MW01096539

What doctors say about . . .
Mommy, I'm Hungry

"Mommy, I'm Hungry" should find its way into the library of mothers who realize that early exposure to good nutrition habits sets the lifetime pattern, yielding lifelong dividends in heightened well-being."
CARLTON FREDERICKS, PH.D., Author, *Nutrition: Your Key to Good Health, Food Facts and Fallacies*

"I think this book simply *must* be in the kitchen of every home where there are children . . . and schools providing lunches should have it on hand when menus are being selected."
GLENN DOMAN, Director, Institutes for the Achievement of Human Potential
Author, *Teach Your Baby to Read* and *What to Do About Your Brain-Injured Child*

"The role of nutrition in health and behavior is far too important to allow our children's choice of foods to be influenced by TV commercials.
"This book details the most practical approach to altering a child's eating habits and establishing proper nutrition."
ALLAN COTT, M.D.
Author, *The Orthomolecular Approach to Learning Disabilities*

"I've practiced pediatrics for over 30 years. And the longer I practice, the more I'm convinced that the road to better health for children doesn't lie in more 'doctoring.' Instead, it relates to changes in life style . . . especially better nutrition.
"*Mommy, I'm Hungry* gives parents who are interested in providing really good food for their children an interesting, comprehensive and practical guide to go by. It is clearly written and should be well received by parents everywhere who are interested in rearing healthier children."
WILLIAM G. CROOK, M.D., The Children's Clinic.
Author, *Are You Allergic?, Your Child and Allergy*

i

Mommy, I'm Hungry

How To Feed Your Child Nutritiously

Patricia McEntire

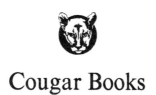

Cougar Books

Published by
Cougar Books
All rights reserved.
Copyright 1982 by Cougar Books
P.O. Box 22246 Sacramento, Ca. 95822

ISBN: 0917982-11-8

Library of Congress Catalog Card No: 79-53202

Edited by Kathleen Campbell Anderson

The excerpt on page 2 is from *Improving Your Child's Behavior Chemistry,*
by Lendon H. Smith, copyright 1976 by Lendon H. Smith. Reprinted
with permission of Prentice-Hall, Inc., Englewood Cliffs, New Jersey.

The recipes on pages 103 and 137 for "dots" and marshmallows are from the
Natural Foods Blender Cookbook by Frieda Nusz, copyright 1966, 1968
and 1972 by Frieda Nusz. Used with the permission of Keats Publishing,
Inc., New Canaan, Connecticut.

The recipe on page 151 for eclairs is reprinted from *The Art of Cooking with
Love and Wheat Germ,* Jane Kinderlehrer, copyright 1977 by Rodale
Press, Inc., Permission granted by Rodale Press, Inc., Emmaus, Pennsyl-
vania.

Printed in the United States of America

9 8 7 6 5 4 3 2 1

To Adelle Davis
who opened the path
to health for me
and to my husband and son
for showing me the way . . .

Special thanks to:

Dr. Carlton Fredericks and Dr. Lendon Smith for their inspiration and genuine interest; Kathleen Anderson for her enthusiasm and editing — without her encouragement this book would not have been written; and to Ruth Pritchard, my publisher, for enduring alongside me the many, many hours and maximum effort to make this book a reality.

Contents

Foreword

I'm delighted with this book. Ms. McEntire has done what I could never do — namely, make good nutrition a practical, easy and fun family affair.

She understands that most of us cannot be changed overnight and has suggestions for *gradualism*. She understands and makes allowances for the vagaries of taste and age-related eating habits. She has been there and knows whereof she speaks.

The book is clear and easy to understand. The message is there for all of us — if you want a loving family free of illness, it is possible.

DR. LENDON H. SMITH, "The Children's Doctor"
Author, *Feed Your Kids Right* and
Improving Your Child's Behavior Chemistry

Introduction

Today many physicians and researchers recognize the role good nutrition plays in health. Many childhood ailments — allergies, hyperactivity, learning disabilities, to name a few — are being linked to poor nutrition and the consumption of sugary foods, chemicals, and additives.

More and more we, as parents, are realizing how essential it is that children receive whole, natural foods. Yet most of us have no idea *how* to go about changing our children's eating habits. This book is about growing nutritionally with our children.

For years, I have worked in close contact with mothers who are searching for ways to help their children eat more healthful food. In teaching them, they have taught me. And I have learned through my son, because we had to reach for answers together.

I hope this book will help you and your family discover a healthy new way of life through truly good nutrition. In today's world it's not always an easy route, but it is a rewarding one. You will need conviction and creativity. Reach for the answers together with your children. If you begin, they will show you the way...

Patricia McEntire
Sacramento, California

A Burst of Light

A new life has burst from your womb. A wondrous world has opened for your child, and, for you, a new beginning. As you hold your little one in your arms for the first time, you wish for your child to be perfect in every way. To meet your child's special needs, you are prepared to give all the warmth, love, and tenderness you are capable of giving. What could be a more satisfying start than nursing your tiny one at your breast, so your newborn may receive the ultimate nourishment *with* your ultimate love?

Breast-Feeding vs. Artificial Food

Breast milk has recently regained acceptance as the most perfect food for babies. Many past misconceptions about breast-feeding have had to be dispelled. Since bodily excretions (urine, feces, sweat) are generally viewed as unclean, breast milk — a secretion — was mistakenly lumped into the same category in many American minds. The fact that the breast is viewed as a sexual object added to people's discomfort: sex and elimination were activities to be performed in private.

Bottle feeding was popular because it was clean and sterile, thought of as an improvement on nature. But the formula in a bottle has never been able to match the food nature provides in the human breast.

Most formulas are a basic mixture of nonfat milk, lactose, coconut and/or soy oil, with some vitamins and minerals added. This basic combination must be diluted with water, since cow's milk has twice the protein of human milk. The mixture must be heated to a high degree to change the large, tough curds into smaller, softer curds. Coconut oil has an extremely high saturated-fat content compared to the low saturated fat content of human milk.

Science has not been able to produce in a formula many of the essential nutrients in breast milk. The balance of those vitamins and minerals which *are* added to a formula is questionable.

A baby uses breast milk with almost 100 percent efficiency, but can utilize only about 50 percent of a formula. This places undue stress on an infant's immature kidneys, since the kidneys must eliminate the proteins and minerals the body cannot use. Frequently, the stress on the infant's body results in severe allergic reactions. The formula is then changed from cow's milk to soy milk, and this often begins a spiral of switching from one formula to another. Each further aggravates the baby's delicate system, so the formula is switched again . . . and again and again.

Here is a typical soy-milk formula: corn syrup, sucrose (sugar), coconut oil, soy oil, soy protein isolate, and water. This formula speaks for itself. It is a mystery to me how any infant could remain healthy on such a sugary, unbalanced concoction.

Since authorities now agree that breast milk is the ultimate food for an infant, why do doctors remain unenthusiastic about breast-feeding? Dr. Lendon H. Smith answers this in his outstanding book, *Improving Your Child's Behavior Chemistry* (© 1976 by Lendon H. Smith, M.D. Published by Prentice-Hall, Inc., Englewood Cliffs, New Jersey 07632).

"Our problem is that if we insist that a mother nurse her baby, and her milk supply is inadequate for some reason, she feels guilty. This discouragement usually cuts the supply further . . . To provide proper protein nutrition we switch the baby to cow's milk, but these are the very babies that so often become allergic to cow's milk.

"The pediatrician is caught between the guilty mother and the allergic baby, so for us to avoid our own uncomfortable stress headaches, we become wishy-washy. 'Try to nurse,' we say, 'but if it's a big drag, use the bottle.' "

In many instances, a male physician is trying to help a new mother in a function they are both unfamiliar with. The study of nutrition and breast-feeding is limited in most medical schools. And, after all, what man has ever nursed a baby?

Moreover, the baby-food industry promotes artificial feeding since millions of dollars profit are involved. The baby-food manufacturer pushes information and samples on doctors and hospitals who, in turn, place the supplemental bottle in the newborn's mouth. The new mother is then sent home with the "emergency" formula, which she uses, and gradually learns to depend upon.

A nursing mother, therefore, should not be completely dependent on doctors for advice. A good place to turn for help is La Leche League, a group of experienced nursing mothers available for advice and support in most cities.

Any woman who feels she cannot nurse her baby because

¶ She doesn't have enough milk or it isn't rich enough
¶ She is afraid her breasts will sag afterward
¶ She wants to lose extra weight gained during pregnancy
¶ She has inverted nipples
¶ She has twins
¶ She has tried unsuccessfully to nurse her other children

may find answers to these and other fears or questions through La Leche League.

Before your baby is born, try to prevent breast-feeding problems from occurring by attending La Leche meetings and reading books on the subject. After your baby is born, La Leche meetings will give you the opportunity to share your feelings, problems, and joys with other mothers.

Your body supplied your baby with what was needed when tucked inside your womb; trust it to supply your baby with the ultimate food after your child is safely in your arms.

New Food

Somewhere between five and seven months old, your little one will be ready for solid food. Start slowly to guard against allergic reactions and to give your baby time to learn how to eat. The first food may be one of the following:

The banana is one of the most popular foods to start with since it is easily digested and causes few allergic reactions.

The avocado, bland and well tolerated, is a powerhouse of vitamins, minerals, protein, and unsaturated fatty acids.

The papaya, a mildly flavored fruit, is easily digested and also aids in the digestion of other foods.

Establishing Solid Food

Your baby's first foods should be of high quality, supplying essential nutrients and not just empty calories.

Feeding your little one nutritious food does not have to be difficult. It is just a matter of having lots of simple foods on hand.

Fruits: Fresh fruit should be selected over frozen (unsweetened) or dried (unsulphured); never use canned unless it is unsweetened. Include unsulfured dried apricots (soaked and put through the blender) liberally as a superior source of iron.

Cheese: Cheese should be mild and soft. Tofu (a very soft, bland cheese made from soybeans) is excellent to start with since it is not made from milk. When you are sure your baby can handle dairy products, try goat cheese, kefir cheese and mild cow-milk cheeses. If available, select raw milk cheeses. Avoid any processed cheeses with chemicals and cheeses which are artificially colored.

Eggs: Eggs should be used if no allergy exists. They are readily absorbed and are one of the highest sources of protein. Use fresh country eggs (or fertile eggs) from chickens that run about and are not stuffed with chemicals.

Nuts and Seeds: Finely ground seeds and nuts are an important source of protein, vitamins, and minerals. They must be fresh, raw, and unsalted. Almonds, pecans, cashews; sunflower, chia, pumpkin, and sesame seeds are good choices for baby's diet. (*Be sure to grind them very fine.*)

Sprouts: This excellent source of nutrients can be grown year round. Liquify sprouts in your blender, add banana and juice for an exciting "salad." Alfalfa sprouts are the most popular.

Milk: Yogurt (without sugar), kefir, buttermilk, and goat's milk add variety to the standard offering of cow's milk.

Fish, Fowl, and Meat: These concentrated proteins should be introduced slowly. Use a variety, but select organ meats over muscle meats. Avoid any meat that contains nitrates or nitrites. (Recent tests have found these preservatives to be highly carcinogenic). Ham, bacon, hot dogs, luncheon meats fit into this category unless purchased at a health food store.

4

Juice: Sources should be fresh squeezed whenever possible. A juice extractor would be a good investment, but is not necessary if raw foods are included in your baby's diet. Orange, apricot, pineapple, papaya, and apple are easily accepted fruit juices, but you might like to try raw carrot mixed with the juices of green vegetables.

Grains: Millet, soy, whole wheat, buckwheat, and brown rice are excellent. Cereal does not have to be a starchy, refined mass, but can supply vital nutrients. Freshly milled raw wheat germ may be used as a cereal or added to other foods to increase their nutritional value. *Hold off on the use of cereals until your baby is ten to twelve months old*; a baby does not yet have the enzymes to properly digest grains.

Sweetening: *Concentrated sweetening should not be fed to any child under one year old.* (This means *no* honey, fructose, maple syrup, raw or refined sugars.)

Nutritional Yeast: This unique food contains a multitude of minerals, B vitamins, and protein. Use only a yeast balanced with calcium and magnesium. (Dr. Donsbach's Yeast 500 is the best tasting.)

Vegetables: Puree any raw vegetables available. When it is necessary to cook vegetables, steam lightly and save the vitamin/mineral-rich liquid to use in soups or other dishes.

Many baby-food cookbooks have recipes for making your own baby food to freeze for later use. This is fine for emergencies or an occasional night out, but I never found it practical. It was important to me that my baby receive raw or fresh cooked food since I prefer the taste and quality of fresh food over canned or frozen in my own diet. Besides, it is quicker to put fresh foods through the blender (or baby-food grinder) than it is to defrost something. And what could be more convenient than giving baby an unseasoned portion of the nutritious dinner you are preparing for the rest of the family?

Suggested Menus and Recipes for Baby's Earliest Meals

BREAKFAST A

Mashed avocado
Scrambled egg
Juice of ½ orange + 1 tsp. nutritional yeast

5

BREAKFAST B

Pureed apricots + 1 tsp. ground raw sesame seeds
Kefir milk

BREAKFAST C

Papaya puree
Plain yogurt + 1 T. ground raw wheat germ
Apricot juice

BREAKFAST D

Ground raw wheat germ + mashed banana + ½ tsp. nutritional
    yeast
Cubes of cheese

BREAKFAST E

Ground nuts and seeds + a few raisins + milk to moisten —
    Grind together
Raw Applesauce*

BREAKFAST F

Cottage cheese + fresh pineapple — *Blend*
Poached egg

LUNCH A

Mashed avocado + 1 T. ground raw almonds
Steamed carrot sticks
Pureed cooked zucchini

LUNCH B

Alfalfa sprouts + banana + fresh orange juice — *Blend*
Cheese omelet with pureed spinach

* Recipe in Chapter Thirteen.

LUNCH C

Potato Salad with Tofu and Cheese*
Baked and pureed acorn squash
Pureed beets

DINNER A

Steamed liver + egg + mashed potato + grated cheese — *Blend*
Steamed pureed rutabagas

DINNER B

1 banana + 3 T. ground raw sunflower seeds + mashed carrot
    — *Blend*
Pureed chicken

DINNER C

Steamed and pureed fish   Cubes of cheese
Pureed asparagus

DESSERTS

This is where the trouble begins. Getting a baby started on desserts is a sure step down the road to the land of goodies. If you feel your child needs extra food, use fruits, Finger Gelatin**, or Honey Custard*, instead of food with empty calories.

Teething Foods

Celery, carrot sticks, peeled apples, peeled pears make excellent teething foods. (Use caution: A chunk could lodge in baby's throat.) A chicken bone (drumstick only) with the gristle removed can be gnawed on for hours.

Teething cookies are not necessary. If you must use them, make your own to insure the purity of ingredients. These cookies may be frozen so they'll feel cold against your baby's gums. Do make sure that your baby is not sensitive to any of the ingredients in the cookie recipe.

* Recipe in Chapter Thirteen.
** Recipe in Chapter Twelve

SUPER TEETHING COOKIES

3 T. unsulphured molasses
2 T. cold-pressed safflower oil
1 egg yolk
¼ cup soy flour
½ cup raw seed flour
¼ cup nutritional yeast
¼ cup carob powder

Mix molasses, oil, and egg yolk. In a separate bowl, mix dry ingredients. Then combine two mixtures to form a stiff dough. Roll out dough, using more soy flour if needed. Press out desired shapes, and bake at 300° for about 25 minutes.

A Word About External Potions

Sometimes we forget that creams and oils we put onto our skin are absorbed into our bodies. It is not a good idea to rub a baby's skin with powders, creams, oils, and lotions that contain mineral oil, chemicals, or other contaminants. The best secret for avoiding diaper rash is to rub the contents of a vitamin E capsule on baby's skin at the first sign of pinkness.

The Most Important of All

The growth you experience with your baby is necessary for a child to mature into a warm, loving, feeling person. Let your little one feel your love: touch, share feelings, exchange laughter and warmth, so your child can develop in a secure and happy environment.

Munchkins on the Run

Somewhere between the ages of one-and-a-half and two, your little explorer will become too independent to be fed by Mommy, although not yet competent with a spoon. The busy toddler spends less time eating, and, consequently, eats smaller amounts. Children this age restrict eating, for the most part, to finger foods and drinks "to go."

Not only do mothers have to contend with this, but many toddlers will eat only one type of food. Most toddlers' eating habits can be broken into three categories:

The Drinker
The Protein Eater
The Carbohydrate Eater

Your child's diet may not fit strictly into one of these categories, but may fluctuate between two or even three of these cycles. Or it may fit staunchly into the same eating pattern day after day.

Whatever your child's food cycle, let the phase run its course. In the meantime, you are challenged with making sure nutritional needs are met. Despite limited choices, you *can* do it — by adding concentrated, nutritious ingredients to those foods your child will accept.

The Drinker

If your little munchkin is a drinker, a bottle probably is close at hand. A bottle is fine, so don't feel guilty if your little one (who was weaned from the breast to a bottle) is still attached to it. In fact, it is an excellent vehicle for nutritious mixtures. The fantastic thing about a bottle or an enclosed cup with a straw is that (1) it doesn't end up on the carpet, and (2) a more concentrated mixture may be accepted since the child's nose isn't in direct contact with the new additions to the diet. If you are using a bottle, use a cross-cut nipple to prevent clogging.

MARVELOUS MUNCHKIN MIX

1 T. carob powder
1 T. honey (less if you can get by with it)
1 egg
1 cup milk (preferably certified raw milk)
1 tsp. safflower oil (cold-pressed with vitamin E added)
½ tsp.-1 T. nutritional yeast
1 T. ground raw sunflower or sesame seeds
1 tsp. soy lecithin

Blend these ingredients together and your toddler will have a superb meal. For a fast snack, freeze this mixture in popsicle molds.

SMOOTHIE

4 or 5 fresh or unsweetened frozen strawberries
½ banana
¼ cup plain yogurt
½ cup fresh orange juice
1 egg
handful of alfalfa sprouts
bit of ice

Blend on high setting until sprouts are completely liquified.

BANANA NUT PLUS

1 cup fresh orange juice
¼ cup plain yogurt
1 T. ground nuts
½ banana
1 tsp. nutritional yeast
1 tsp. lecithin

Blend until smooth.

QUICK DYNAMITE

1 cup milk (preferably certified raw)
½ banana
1 egg
1 T. of Naura Hayden's Dynamite Shake Mix (yeast, lecithin,
   nonfat milk powder, vitamins, and minerals) or Dr. Donsbach Glan-Pro protein powder
1 T. carob powder

Blend until smooth.

This drink is a lifesaver for the harried housewife or working
Mommy, but it is more expensive than if you buy yeast and
lecithin separately.

JUICY DELIGHT

½ cup fresh carrot juice
½ cup coconut juice (Lakewood [brandname] makes one
   without sugar)
¼ cup pineapple juice
¼ cup papaya juice
1 egg
1 tsp. nutritional yeast
1 tsp. soy protein
bit of ice

Blend until ice is crushed.

The Protein Eater

The protein eater will need lots of variation. Offer many
kinds of protein foods, not just meat. Include a generous supply
of ground nuts and seeds, fish, chicken, organ meats, and
various cheeses, but offer these foods after or in conjunction
with fruits and vegetables.

The protein eater can really restrict your freedom to
experiment with new combinations of food. A child in the
protein cycle may go to such extremes as separating the meat
sauce from the spaghetti. This is no cause for alarm. Your child
may be purposely avoiding allergenic foods, so go easy on the
addition of any grains or flour to the diet.

Tuna, Chicken, or Egg Salad with Pizzazz

Tuna, chicken, or egg salad does not have to be protein and mayonnaise with a bit of celery thrown in once in a while. It can be different each time you make it, and can offer a wide spectrum of nutrients. Try adding:

grated carrot	avocado
celery	tofu (soy cheese)
sprouts	cheese
ground raw nuts and seeds	egg (to tuna or chicken)

Mayonnnaise should be homemade* or purchased at a health food store. Try substituting plain yogurt for ¼ of the mayonnaise.

Meat Loaf or Hamburger Supreme

Instead of using plain ground beef and bread crumbs, power-pack your meat loaf with some of the following:

Meat
ground liver
ground heart
Start with a small amount of organ meat and work up slowly to about ¼ lb. to every ¾ lb. ground beef.

Breading
raw wheat germ
Fearn [brand name] Sesame Burger Mix
raw ground seeds or nuts

Additions
grated vegetables, such as carrots and zucchini
egg
nutritional yeast

Flavorings
tomato sauce
thyme
basil
kelp
ketchup made with honey

---

* Recipe in Chapter Thirteen.

THE UN-SANDWICH

Use slices of fruits, vegetables, or cheese as the "bread" of the sandwich and the filling may be nut or seed butters, cheese, proteins (tuna, chicken, egg), fruits or vegetables.

The Bread

banana slices or chips
apple slices
lettuce leaves (rolled)
cucumber slices
cheese slices
carrot slices
pear slices
beet slices
celery
zucchini

The Filling

peanut butter
raw cheddar cheese
cottage cheese and pineapple
tuna salad
egg salad
avocado
almond butter
kefir cheese or cream cheese
chicken salad
apple

You may serve these Un-Sandwiches open-faced or cut up into bite-cubes. Invent your own. Mommies watching their weight will enjoy the Un-Sandwich too!

The Carbohydrate Eater

My son fits perfectly into this category. Bread, muffins, cookies, pancakes — he devours them all! I struggled with various methods to get more protein into him, to no avail. In desperation one day, I replaced the flour in a cookie recipe with nutritional yeast, powdered milk, wheat germ, ground seeds, and soy powder. Surprisingly, the neighborhood children, as well as my son, gobbled up the "cookies deluxe" and asked for more. I began experimenting and found that decreasing flour and increasing high protein substances didn't alter the taste!

Any recipe that does not require a great deal of rising can be altered by changing each cup of sugar into ¾ cup honey; substituting more nutritious ingredients for at least ½ of the flour; and using whole grain flour for the remaining flour, increasing the quantity by ¼ cup. Decrease the oven temperature by about 25 degrees.

For example, a recipe calls for:

1 cup sugar
½ cup butter   ¼ tsp. salt
2 eggs

½ tsp. vanilla
1½ cups white flour
2 tsp. baking powder

Boost it nutritionally by changing it to something like this:

¾ cup honey
½ cup butter
2 eggs
½ tsp. pure vanilla
½ cup whole wheat pastry flour
¼ cup non-instant milk powder
½ cup raw sunflower seed flour
2 T. nutritional yeast
2 T. protein powder
2 tsp. low-sodium baking powder

This approach makes it easy to get protein into your little one's diet. But don't forget about raw fruits and vegetables. Make these foods exciting; don't stick to apples, oranges, and carrots. If, by chance, your child rejects all raw food, try offering him natural milkshakes or popsicles made from freshly blended fruits and vegetables.

Gingerbread Munchkins

½ cup whole wheat pastry flour
½ cup ground raw wheat germ
½ cup non-instant milk powder
1½ cups raw seed or nut flour
1 T. nutritional yeast
1 tsp. ginger
¼ tsp. cinnamon
¼ tsp. nutmeg
½ cup cold-pressed safflower oil
½ cup unsulfured molasses

Mix dry ingredients. Combine oil and molasses and add to dry ingredients. Roll out to about ⅜ of an inch thick, dusting with soy flour as needed. Press out with gingerbread-man cookie cutter. Add facial features with nuts, seeds, or raisins. Bake for about 30 minutes at 300°.

Power Pancakes

¼ cup buckwheat or whole wheat flour
1 T. nutritional yeast
½ cup seed or nut flour
2 tsp. baking soda
1 egg
1 cup plain yogurt or milk
3 T. melted butter

Combine dry ingredients. Add mixed wet ingredients, stirring quickly. Add milk if too thick.

Foods for Fingers

Little munchkins are so busy discovering new things that they don't want to be bothered using a fork or spoon. They love finger food because they can eat it on the run. The diet is simplified with finger foods, but it can lead to the use of empty foods like crackers, cookies, and chips. Keep lots of nutritious tidbits on hand. Fruits, vegetables, fish, chicken, meat, cheese, or foods made from some of the recipes in the last chapter of this book can insure proper nutrients for your active toddler.

Ideas for Nutritious Tidbits:

cheese
chunks of fresh fruit
cooked garbanzo beans
cubes of meat/chicken/turkey
dried fruit
frozen fruit
frozen peas or grapes

Fruit Leather Rolls*
Honey Bran Muffins*
raw vegetables with dip*
Seed Crackers*
shrimp
slices of avocado
sprouts

* Recipes in Chapter Thirteen.

Con-Cen-Tration

Getting your child to eat enough good food at any age can be quite a challenge. The easiest way to get your child to accept good food, of course, would be to start feeding the right food at birth. Needless to say, most people find out too late how to feed themselves properly, let alone their children.

Changing your family's eating habits is not something that will happen overnight. It is a slow, gradual learning process, fraught with backsliding. The key to getting your family to adopt healthful eating habits is the example you set yourself.

Learn to deal with situations immediately, instead of postponing that difficult "no" to another time. Young children can accept "no" (though not always graciously, which is to be expected), and they can accept "yes." But they cannot accept the unstable concept of "sometimes" or "maybe."

Acceptance of a proper diet is difficult if you tell your child in one breath that sugar destroys B vitamins and, in the next, say that eating a little bit of sugar won't hurt "just this once." Very young children find it especially frustrating and confusing when Mommy says it's okay to have sugar cookies one day, but not the next. Why should it be acceptable just on those days when Mother gives in?

A drink of cola, a sugary cookie, or a mound of ice cream won't do much damage once in a while. What does do the damage is your tolerance of it. And "just this once" tends to proliferate as vacations, parties, and outings pop up.

As children grow older, they gradually learn to accept "sometimes" and "maybe." They will have been taught which foods are the most satisfying to eat and will have acquired a taste for them. Also, they will have learned to plan ahead so they can deal effectively with difficult situations on their own.

There is a physical as well as emotional adjustment to a change in diet. Pushing someone too fast can make them quickly lose interest, as I ruefully learned. My own experience in changing someone's eating habits started with my husband. My husband is open to a lot of things, but when I prepared our first meal and set a bowl of vitamins before him, he was quite blunt.

"I won't take a bowlful of vitamins."

At first there were remarks like, "What is *that*?", "Isn't that expensive?", "I just can't give up my rocky-road ice cream", and "O-o-o-oo, donuts!"

Even Daddies need pampering with their diet at times! Remaining patient with his bouts of cola, candy, and especially donuts, I found these cravings for sugar gradually lessened as his body gained the nutrients it really craved.

The more sugar you eat, the more B vitamins you waste and the more B vitamins you waste, the more sugar you crave. Thus, you become bound in a vicious cycle that is difficult to break. It isn't easy to avoid refined sugar since sugar is hidden in so many strange places — ketchup, salt, salad dressings, potato chips, and packaged dinner mixes — to name a few. Even if you do not buy the obvious sugar-laden goodies (such as cookies, cereals, cake, candy), your family can be ingesting quite a bit of sugar without knowing it.

To simply remove sugar from the diet is not always possible because of physical addiction. In the transition process of removing sugar from the diet, you must use high-quality, concentrated foods in order to overcome the deficiencies caused by empty food.

Concentrated foods come in many forms and can be used in a multitude of ways. Some may be new to you, but, with a bit of experimenting, you can learn to include these concentrated foods in your favorite recipes.

Concentrated Foods

Nutritional Yeast: The most important addition you can make to any recipe. Because it is very concentrated, 1 or 2 tablespoons is sufficient. Start out with 1 teaspoon and work up to more. If you are deficient in B vitamins, gas may form in your stomach unless you start out slowly. Add yeast to any breadstuff without change of flavor.

Desiccated Liver Powder: A potent addition, best used in tiny amounts because of the strong taste. Add to tomato juice or meat loaf (as well as using fresh ground liver in the loaf).

Seed Flour: Mild-tasting seed or nut flour you can grind yourself (in blender or grinder) from whole raw seeds or nuts. Can replace ½ of flour in cookies or muffins.

Sprouts: A replacement for lettuce that can be used in salads, gelatin molds, blender drinks, or even muffins.

Fruits and Vegetables: Grated vegetables can be added to practically anything! Dried fruits are tasty snacks.

Wheat Germ: Raw wheat germ can be used as a cereal by itself or as an addition to another cereal. Grind wheat germ to a fine texture and use as a flour or to boost homemade snacks.

Lecithin: As a powder it can be used in blender drinks or in baking.

Kelp: A good seasoning, but strong tasting, so use in tiny amounts.

Protein powder: High quality protein powder may be used to replace ¼ cup flour in recipes.

Rice Polish: A substitute for flour in baking.

Soy Flour: A substitute for flour, with two precautions. (1) It browns more quickly during baking than wheat flour. (2) The batter will have a raw taste that disappears after baking.

Non-Instant Milk Powder: Milk or whey powder also will cause baked goods to brown faster. Add to just about anything without a change in taste.

Arrowroot: A thickening agent that can take the place of cornstarch. One tablespoon will thicken one cup of liquid.

Questions may be forming in your mind about what some of these foods are and if they are harmful or really necessary.

All of these are natural foods, or derivatives of natural foods, that contain high quantities of vitamins and minerals. You need not use them all every day, but they should be liberally included in your family's daily diet to provide essential nutrients missing from the average American diet.

What these foods are and what each offers nutritionally is discussed in more detail in Chapter Twelve.

Choosing

The ingredients you introduce to your family will vary according to individual needs. If your child consumes large quantities of milk or cheese, milk powder will not be needed in cookies or cake; instead you may use seed flour, wheat germ, and nutritional yeast. In cases where children are allergic to milk or wheat, other concentrated foods should be substituted for milk powder and wheat germ. Remember, an allergic child does not necessarily react with a rash, but may react with hyperactivity, exhaustion, colds, headaches, nausea, etc. If you suspect an allergy, try eliminating the more common allergens (wheat, milk, eggs) to find out what your child is sensitive to.

Concentrated foods are not harmful, but must be chosen carefully. Nutritional yeast and lecithin are high in phosphorus and must be purchased with balanced minerals. Protein powder must be of high quality and *not* contain sugar and/or chemicals.* Wheat germ must be freshly milled; if you don't plan to use it within a few weeks' time, keep it frozen. Seed flour needs to be refrigerated as soon as it is ground. Any organ meats purchased should be from animals raised naturally. (Otherwise, the organs have filtered and accumulated many chemicals.) Try to obtain the freshest, purest food available, and store it in tightly sealed containers, refrigerating when necessary.

Beginning

No one is able to change their eating patterns in a day, or a month, or even six months. Most of us carry into adulthood our emotional needs for sugar. We pass on to our children the idea of sugar as reward and help them establish a physical craving for it.

At first, you may have to sneak these concentrated foods into recipes when no one is looking. Meanwhile, help your child to understand what a body needs to function properly. When your child has come to accept the new changes in diet, you can explain what you add to increase the nutritional value of cookies

---

* Trophic Lecithin, Dr. Donsbach Yeast 500, Dr. Donsbach Glan-pro Protein powder and Naura Hayden's Dynamite powder are good choices.

or meat loaf as you are making it. The best time to talk about nutrition is when your child asks.

Children may enjoy helping in the kitchen. Let them experiment. It's usually worth the mess. For example, my son refuses to drink nutritional yeast mixed with juice, but will eat it by the tablespoon if permitted to do it himself while helping me cook. If you have ever tasted nutritional yeast, you realize how incredible it is that he could eat it in this fashion! Yet, each of us is unique in our likes and dislikes, and children should be given the freedom to find out what tastes best to them, in what form. Cooking with Mommy or Daddy helps your child to accept the taste and smell of natural ingredients.

Yeast, lecithin, and powdered milk should become common pantry shelf items, as white flour, sugar, and salt once were. Let your child accept nutritional foods as okay foods to have around, and learn to ingest these new foods — physically and emotionally.

The Name of the Game

Waiting in the checkout lane at the supermarket, I am always disturbed to see the number of baskets filled with white bread, sugar cereals, TV dinners, soda pop, candy, potato chips, flavored gelatin, cake mixes, canned spaghetti, luncheon meats, canned vegetables, instant drink mixes, and all kinds of other processed foods. I find it hard to resist tapping the mother on the shoulder and asking her how she can possibly buy these empty foods for her children *and think she is feeding them well.* Are we so well trained as consumers that we believe everything the media feeds us?

Next time you hear one of these advertising slogans, stop to think about it.

"Good for You!" — Sugar cereals may contain as much sugar as candy, as well as coloring, flavoring, and preservatives.

"No Preservatives" — A deceiving claim since sugar, artificial color, and artificial flavor are frequently added to these products.

"Vitamin C Added" — What they don't tell you is that the body needs every bit (and sometimes more) of that Vitamin C to detoxify the poisonous chemicals in this artificially colored and flavored sugar water.

"Kids Love It!" — Why not just hand them the sugar bowl? It's much cheaper. The taste kids supposedly love is sugar. But it isn't that they love it; they are addicted to it.

"Gives Your Spirits a Lift" — And your pancreas a jolt!

"Tastes Like the Real Thing" — Can you believe two percent real maple syrup? Sugar, corn syrup, carmel color, and artificial flavorings make up the other 98 percent.

"10 Percent Real Fruit Juice" — Who could possibly want 10 percent juice in a 90 percent base of sugar, water, and artificial color and flavor?

"They're So Fresh!" — We are so concerned about freshness and purity (pure white sugar and flour) that we have stripped our food of nutrients. Freshness is important, but if the food does not contain any nutrients, it matters little whether it is fresh or not. Adding two or three B vitamins to a mixture of white sugar and flour is a worthless gesture since the sugar in the product will far outweigh the benefit.

The real clincher is:
"Without Chemicals Life Itself Would Be Impossible" — But the body chemistry of a human being is upset by the introduction of *foreign* chemicals. The result can be serious physical and emotional disorders.

Is the Name of the Game M-O-N-E-Y?

It is difficult for me to believe that any person would sacrifice the health of a nation for the almighty dollar. Yet, the number of health-destroying products on the market is growing. The only other explanation is that the manufacturers of these products don't believe there is any relation between eating correctly and the degree of health one has.

When I was a child, my family had a beautiful German Shepherd. I can remember my father reprimanding me for feeding candy to the dog.

"Good dogs should never have sweets. It will ruin their health."

My father simply did not see the same association with his own or his children's health, although he certainly loved us and wanted the very best for us. Maybe the same is true for many food companies. They simply don't see — or don't want to see — the relationship between food and health.

One of the problems here is that people often think only in terms of *minimal* health. We tend to waver from black to white — either you have good health or you do not — there are no in-

23

betweens. Is the line between disease and health really that
defined? If you don't have scurvy, you have met your requirements for Vitamin C to the very minimum. But that does not
mean you have achieved a maximum state of health which can
prevent other, less drastic ailments. People do not die on the
spot from ingesting large quantities of refined sugar and
chemical preservatives . . . but that does not mean it is good for
them!

As long as there are misconceptions about what the body
needs to function properly and to achieve maximum health,
processed foods will be big business. Businesses will continue to
make huge profits if they and the public are persuaded that no
harm is being done. That is why food companies contribute
heavily to research in nutrition.

Some "prominent" researchers do insist that high amounts
of refined sugars, chemical additives, artificial coloring and
flavoring are not harmful. But since processed food companies
contribute heavily to this research their products can hardly be
denounced as harmful.

Our children are paying the real price. Why should we
permit ourselves to buy what big business promotes, knowing
that it is more interested in profits than in our children's well-
being?

Additives — "Minute Amounts of Tested Chemicals"

Here are the two usual arguments that chemicals added to
foods are perfectly safe:

"Additives Have Been Tested" — The amount of money
required for testing the effects of chemicals is incredible, not to
mention the amount of time required for long term and
cumulative effects. The most serious problem, though, is that
these chemicals cannot be tested in combination with each
other, since the various combinations found in foods are endless.
The chemicals in a candy bar may be found to be harmless, but
we do not know what happens when that candy bar is eaten at
the same time as a hot dog with mustard.

*"Additives Are Added to Foods in Minute Amounts and
Pass Right through the Body without Causing any Harm"* — A
healthy person is capable of throwing off small amounts of
poisonous substances that invade the body. The fact is, our

bodies are so overwhelmed by chemical poisons in our food, water, and air that we cannot rid ourselves of them. Adding a little bit of posion may seem unimportant. Even though chemicals are measured in parts per million, they do not belong in the body, and it is not known what amounts are passed right through or stored in the fatty tissue of our bodies.

Adding chemicals to our food supply may not immediately kill us, but there are lots of in-between results such as allergies, hyperactivity, headaches, fatigue, nausea, mental disorders. The cumulative effect of all these chemicals bombarding our bodies is increasingly more severe problems. Before long, if diets aren't changed, there will be even more serious, life-threatening reactions.

The Sugar Trap

The conflicting opinions held by the health experts cause so much confusion that many people sovle their "sugar dilemma" by adopting the attitude, "What I'm eating hasn't killed me yet, so it must be O.K." Of course, it is practically impossible to avoid sugar consumption if one shops in an ordinary supermarket, because packaged products are so heavily laced with it.

We have all heard the statements that sugar gives you energy. The consumption of refined sugar does *jolt* us with a sugar "high" — an immediate rise in blood sugar level. This, in turn, causes the pancreas to release insulin, necessary to combat the dangerously high level of sugar in the bloodstream. Frequent jolting (overstimulation) with refined sugar is damaging since it will not only cause the pancreas to overreact (by producing too much insulin), but will eventually cause the pancreas to lose its ability to release the correct amount of insulin for metabolism of carbohydrates.

To make matters worse, the digestion of refined sugar, devoid of any nutrients itself, depletes the body's vitamin-mineral reserves.

Which Sweetening Do You Choose for Your Child?

Sweetening comes in many forms, from dangerous to nutritious. Know your sweetenings and choose for your child only those that enhance health, not cripple it.

White Sugar: Sugar stripped of all nutrients, except empty calories. Usually derived from sugar cane or sugar beet. Causes high-low blood sugar fluctuations due to its severe stress on the body.

Brown Sugar: White sugar with molasses added. Causes exactly the same reaction that white sugar does, but, because of the molasses, it contains a miniscule amount of nutrients.

Raw Sugar: Unbleached sugar with minute amounts of nutrients left in. Usually represented as turbinado sugar. Causes same reaction as white sugar does, but has a few nutrients.

Yellow D Sugar: Raw sugar with molasses added that causes blood sugar fluctuations.

Date Sugar: Sugar derived from crystallized dates. Not as concentrated as other sugars, but too sweet for many people.

Coconut Sugar: Ground, unsweetened coconut is an acceptable substitute for powdered sugar.

Fructose: Sugar derived not from fruit as popularly thought, but from corn or beets. Has same appearance as white sugar and is about twice as sweet. Does not cause immediate fluctuations in blood sugar levels, but it does not contain enough nutrients to build health. Too concentrated to use very often.

Barley, Rice, or Wheat Syrup: Derived from grains. Can be used occasionally, but too sweet for some people.

Real Maple Syrup: An expensive sweetening derived from the sap of maple trees. May be used occasionally for change of taste. Grade C contains the highest concentration of nutrients.

Raw, Unfiltered Honey: An invert, predigested sweetening that is easily assimilated. Contains quality nutrients. Made up of two sugars: 40 percent dextrose and 60 percent levulose. Levulose does not cause fluctuations in the blood sugar level. Tupelo honey contains the highest level of levulose and should be used exclusively for those with low blood sugar.

Blackstrap Molasses: Very nutritious sweetener, but strong taste limits its use. Blackstrap molasses is the cane syrup thrown off in the last spinning of the sugar refining process.

Eating naturally sweet foods eliminates high-low blood sugar fluctuations. The digestion of an apple or a glass of milk takes much longer, so the natural sugar is slowly introduced into the system. Honey (or molasses) is much more concentrated than whole, natural fruit, so it should definitely be used in moderation. Eliminating it entirely, however, is not very feasible in our culture.

Learning To Live Without Sugar

We can try to raise our children without the sugar-reward syndrome, but we cannot protect them from what they encounter outside the home. They will see and hear the kinds of sugar promotion discussed in this chapter. They will see friends and adults indulging in sugar consumption.

We can teach our children to deal with these outside influences by preparing snacks and desserts that build health, so they will not feel deprived or different. The addition of nutritious substances (such as nutritional yeast, ground seeds, wheat germ, etc.) to desserts will not only build health, but will eliminate the craving for sugar (an addiction caused by nutrient deficiencies) that so many of us are shackled with.

You and your family will gradually lose desire for sugar as your eliminate it from your diet. Foods that are heavily sweetened will more and more often taste too sweet. My son Shawn, at four, was so sensitive to hidden sugar that I learned from his observations.

One day Shawn became hungry for a snack while we were out shopping. We combed a health food store, found some "natural" carrot cake and bought it for him. In anticipation, he held the cellophane wrapped cake up to his nose and smelled.

"Mommy, this cake has sugar in it. I don't want it."

It had never occurred to me that it was possible to *smell* the presence of refined sugar in baked goods. I sniffed it myself — and, sure enough! Even through the wrapping, I could detect it too.

Dealing with the Chemical-Sugar Industry

When we buy a product that is devoid of nutrients, or one that is heavily laced with sugar and/or chemicals, we are promoting a product. We are telling the manufacturer, in effect, that the product is acceptable. If it sells it has to be good! If we refuse to buy the sugary, chemical-laden foods, they will no longer be produced, since they exist only for profit. This overpowering surge of poisons into our food supply is rapidly increasing as we accept convenience as a worthwhile substitute for good health.

Bouncing Off the Walls

Our children are changing. Allergies, sickness, deviant behavior, learning disabilities, hypoglycemia, and mental disorders are far too prevalent today. Is it surprising so many children react to the chemical feast by bouncing off walls?

To control these abnormalities, the usual methods range anywhere from drugs to behavior modification to psychotherapy to special schools to nothing at all (the child will outgrow it). These methods mask the symptoms; they don't cure the problem.

Something is causing these disorders, yet authorities can't seem to agree on what the something is. There are those who insist that diet has nothing to do with the multitude of disorders that plague our children. (In the case of physical injury to the brain this is true.) Then there are those who do recognize these disorders as a reaction to some, or all, of the following:

¶ Artificial colors, flavors, and preservatives.
¶ Refined sugar and flour.
¶ Severe deficiencies of nutrients.
¶ Allergies to food and/or inhalants.
¶ Toxins in our air, water, and food.

All the parts of the puzzle have been found, but no one seems able to put them together. Those who view artificial colors and flavors as a threat to our children don't seem to recognize the effects sugar has; and those who see the importance of vitamins tend to ignore the minerals, and on it goes.

Even if the unresolved causes of these disorders were all put together and finally understood, we would still be faced with *how* to change the eating habits of our children. Many authorities find it easy to say *change* the diet, but do not find it as easy to say *how* to go about it.

While we are waiting around for the authorities to get together on just what is causing all the disorders in our children — *our children are getting worse.*

Instead of masking the symptoms or pretending that our children will outgrow their disorders, let's face these abnormal reactions in our children. Let's attempt to understand what many of us have to deal with, and what many more of us will face.

Our Hyperactive Children

Hyperactivity is probably the most well-known disorder that affects our children. There are few of us that do not know a hyperactive child. Of course, knowing one and having to deal with one are entirely different things. Hyperactivity causes a tremendous drain on the parents, and, in desperation, they will choose the quickest method possible (that their doctor suggests) to control the situation.

The usual method is a stimulant. Obviously, something is terribly twisted in the child's chemistry if stimulants have a sedative effect. With the physician's support, the parents continue the drug method, believing there is no other effective way to stop hyperactivity. The parents are left with the guilt of giving their child a drug, not to cure, but to control.

A fresh approach in dealing with hyperactivity is the Feingold Diet, developed by Dr. Benjamin Feingold at the Kaiser-Permanente Medical Center, San Francisco. This diet removes artificial colors and flavors and several fruits from the child's diet. The Feingold Diet is a tremendous step in the right direction. But with all due respect to Dr. Feingold, it is not complete. Large amounts of sugar persist in the diet, and the necessity of vitamins and minerals is overlooked.

Hyperactivity is often intertwined with allergy and hypoglycemia in a frightening way. All three disorders seem to react off one another, sometimes resulting in a hyperactive, allergic, hypoglycemic child. Thus, hyperactivity is often a *reaction* resulting from allergy and/or hypoglycemia.

Our Allergic Children

Adelle Davis, a pioneer in the field of nutrition, described allergic responses as the body's inability to properly break down foods due to an insufficient supply of digestive juices and enzymes. She believed that allergies result when substances formed from partially digested foods act as irritants to the body because they pass into the blood in abnormally large particles.

A deficiency of B vitamins, in particular, decreases production of enzymes and digestive juices. This in turn leads to incomplete digestion, which can result in allergies, according to Davis' theory.

The surge of chemicals and high-sugar foods does often overpower our bodies, causing deficiencies, and making our normal bodily processes unable to function as they should.

Allergy often begins as a pattern in infancy when the infant is switched from one formula to another until one is found that the infant can tolerate. There have been instances where no suitable formula can be found, so human milk is used to save the infant's life. It would save a lot of time, effort, and health if we all nursed our infants, when able, instead of needlessly exposing them to the threat of allergic reactions.

Allergic responses are closely linked to hypoglycemia. Often hypoglycemia cannot be controlled until allergic foods are removed from the diet. Allergic foods tend to be the foods a child eats a great deal of such as milk, wheat, egg, sugar, corn, citrus.

An allergic reaction is specific to each person. Some children do not react with the more common symptoms (such as wheezing, hives, hay fever, runny nose, rash), but with fatigue, nausea, depression, hyperactivity, headaches, or whatever their specific reaction is.

Cornering the allergens and eliminating them controls the allergic responses, but this is not the final solution when chemical inhalants are involved. I believed that avoiding specific allergic substances cured allergies until I met a young man who was allergic to virtually everything. I thought this was almost unheard of — to be so allergic to your environment it is a horrendous struggle just to exist. He could not:

¶ Read without falling asleep because of allergy to the ink.

¶ Work without becoming depressed because of allergies to chemicals used in cleaning solutions and insecticides present in most work environments.

¶ Drive without delayed reactions because of allergy to the exhaust.

¶ Eat without feeling nauseous because of allergies to the toxins in the food supply.

¶ Walk without disorientation because of allergy to pollen, exhaust fumes, or pollutants in the air.

¶ Live without utter frustration because of allergy to dust, rugs, gas, paint, and a multitude of other items normally found in a home.

Meeting this young man was just the beginning of what I was to learn, because I discovered he is not the only person like this. Thankfully, there are clinical ecologists (physicians interested in the study of man's reaction to his environment) who can uncover allergies mediated by specific food, inhalant, and chemical exposures. But the list of such crippling allergic reactions is endless — and the number of people affected is ever-growing. As I talk to the parents of highly sensitive children, and to the affected people themselves, a wave of fear rushes through me — *is this just the beginning of what is to come?*

Our Hypoglycemic Children

The large number of people who are now being diagnosed as hypoglycemic (low blood sugar) has caused skeptics to call it a fad disease. The symptoms of this disease once caused physicians to recommend a psychiatrist. (Some still do.) It was thought to be all in the mind, since there didn't appear to be anything physically wrong. When hypoglycemia was recognized, many doctors recommended eating candy bars. (Some still do.) It seemed logical to assume that eating sugar would raise the blood sugar level. The results were disastrous.

Hypoglycemia is a condition in which the body produces too much insulin. Eating sugar *increases* insulin-production, which results in *lower* blood sugar. This aggravates rather than improves the hypoglycemic (low blood sugar) condition.

Back at the drawing board, experts decided that high protein would control low blood sugar. This worked pretty well, but some of the experts got a little out of hand. They started recommending huge quantities of protein with a few vegetables and some oil, thus avoiding milk products, fruits, juices, and grains.

31

There are as many types of hypoglycemia as there are the people who have it. Each of us is unique and so are our requirements for nutrients. Complete vegetarianism is too starchy for a hypoglycemic to metabolize; a diet too extreme in protein overloads a child's system.

We need to help our children achieve the fine balance that supplies correct amounts of protein, raw fruits and vegetables, fats, and grains. Keep a close watch on the physical and emotional state of your child until the correct food balance is found. Anxiety, nervousness, exhaustion, irritability, insomnia, hyperactivity, headaches, depression, and "a cold that just doesn't go away"are a few of the more common responses children have to hypoglycemia and the hidden allergies that may accompany it. You can pinpoint these responses to what is being eaten if only whole unprocessed foods are ingested.

Concentrated sweeteners and starches (such as noodles, legumes, grains, bread) should be avoided until you have an idea how much carbohydrate the child can comfortably handle.

When the carbohydrate level is fairly well established, introduce starchy foods in meals with protein and fat. This slows down the digestion of carbohydrates, keeping blood sugar on an even keel.

Resolving sugar/starch addictions that hypoglycemics suffer is a relearning process; it takes *time*. Superior food will shorten the length of time considerably. Severely afflicted hypoglycemics will require additional high doses of nutrients as well as close inspection for allergenic foods that may be perpetuating the allergic-hypoglycemic response.

Our Children with Learning Disabilities

The number of children with learning disabilities in this country is appalling. Fortunately, children with learning disabilities are now recognized, instead of being labeled underachievers or retarded as they were in the past. Still, there is no cure for children with learning disabilities, only remedial help in the form of special education.

There are as many types and degrees of learning disabilities as there are allergies. The brain may respond allergically just as any system of the body may react. Thus mood, memory, perception, comprehension may be altered due to an allergic - hypoglycemic response.In balancing the child's diet as recommended, learning problems also may be alleviated if the biochemical cause can be determined.

Our Children with Poor Health

Many of our children fall into this category — those who experience constipation, frequent colds, infections, flu, acne, fatigue, and, basically, never seem quite well. These are the children whose diet is not supplying them with the proper nutrients to remain healthy. They are not sick enough to cause any alarm, but their bodies are putting out signals that something is not quite right.

Our Schizophrenic Children

Othomolecular psychiatry is replacing the concept of emotional disturbance with that of chemical disturbance. Conventional treatments for schizophrenia (psychotherapy, shock treatment, and drug therapy) are losing their foothold as research discovers the important influence of body chemistry on the mind.

Abnormal requirements for vitamins/minerals, allergic reponses, hypoglycemia, and/or faulty nutrition may all be related sources of a haywire body chemistry that results in schizophrenia. Finding and eliminating these sources requires:

¶ Thorough searching for possible allergies — with internal and/or external causes.

¶ A superior diet,

¶ A doctor who can recommend the proper dosages of nutrients.

Despite findings relating schizophrenia to nutrient deficiencies and other body dysfunctions, there are still many severely disturbed children sitting in mental hospitals in drugged silence. Many more children in homes across the country are deprived of the joys of childhood while experts grope for answers. Isn't it time for us to try to find some answers through our own children, but using methods that are natural and harmless? Even Sigmund Freud, the father of psychoanalysis, believed that schizophrenia might someday be traced to physical causes, and, therefore, the cure would also lie in organic treatment. Freud wrote:

"All our provisional ideas in psychology will some day be based on organic structure. This makes it probable that special substances and special chemicals control the operation."

Our Autistic Children

The treatment for autistic children most often is behavior modification. Imagine a hyperactive child or a child with a learning disability being *forced* to become *normal*, even though they are unable to do so. Behavior modification doesn't work very well, but it is still the most common approach taken with autistic children.

The total answer to helping the autistic child has not been discovered, but fulfilling your child's nutritional requirements, uncovering allergies, trying optimal dosages of vitamins and minerals under a doctor's care is definitely a step in the right direction.

Dr. Carl C. Pfeiffer writes in his excellent book, *Zinc and Other Micro-Nutrients* (Pivot 1978), "Zinc is important in the retina and a lack of zinc makes direct vision painful; thus the child uses his peripheral vision to greet visitors." Zinc is just the tip of the iceberg since the autistic child needs a total approach to health — but it is a *beginning* . . .

Our Sick and Diseased Children

We hear of children with arthritis, cancer, kidney disease, and other frightening diseases; sometimes we are even involved with such children. But when illness strikes your own child — as happened to me — it is different. It is an unexpected nightmare from which there seems no escape.

Suddenly, your child is completely in the hands of a physician. Qualified? Yes, but not in the field of nutrition. If you should venture to mention the use of vitamins and minerals in curing your child, the physician is apt to either grow hostile or be highly amused. Nevertheless, we follow the physician's orders without question. The doctor certainly is a skilled practitioner and is sincerely trying to help. We are also terribly frightened; more than anything, we want our child to be well.

Medically, the physician knows exactly what should be done — from the standpoint of both knowledge and experience. Nutritionally, the doctor knows very little. The parents are torn — trusting the physician medically, but realizing his knowledge of nutrition is inadequate.

Nutritionally oriented physicians are difficult to find. The study of nutrition must be done on one's own, and not many physicians like to rock the boat by using techniques different from what they were taught in medical school. This leaves our children to be treated with drugs, which sometimes relieve sickness and sometimes do not.

In my opinion, many afflictions that kill or cripple our children are not mysterious ills. They are nutritional crimes against our children.

Our Brain-Injured Children

When our son Shawn was 27 months old, he climbed to the top of a slide and fell six feet onto a cement surface.

The ensuing nightmare was one of screaming, X-rays, intensive care, blood tests, injections, a brain scan, crying, an arteriogram, I.V.s, drugs, paralysis, and emotions torn to pieces. The final diagnosis was that the fall had caused a stroke that paralyzed the entire left side of our son's body. There was very little chance that he would ever return to normal.

It can happen just that fast. A high fever, being struck by a car, revival after near-drowning, convulsions, trauma during or before birth, and hundreds of other factors can cause brain cells to be destroyed by a lack of oxygen, resulting in irreparable injury to brain function. When brain cells are dead they are dead, and it is believed that they cannot be reactivated. It matters little how the injury occurred, only how much damage occurred and what will be done about it.

Medical science is terribly inadequate in dealing with injury to the brain. Sometimes the physician can stop further injury. The physician can usually identify where and to what extent the injury occurs. But there is not much medical doctors can do in the way of curing the existing injury.

In our case, it was fortunate that I was knowledgeable in the field of nutrition and familiar with brain-injured children, having once worked closely with a cerebral palsied child. The parents of that child had applied the intense therapy of The Institutes for the Achievement of Human Potential to stimulate neurological growth in their son.

The Institutes has had significant success in rehabilitating brain-injured children. A small group of professionals (a brain surgeon, a psychologist, a psychiatrist also trained as a physical therapist, a speech therapist, an educator, and a nurse) formed The Institutes for the Achievement of Human Potential when they realized that traditional methods were ineffecive in curing brain-injured children. They developed a therapy which stimu-lates brain cells to take on new functions.

Among other factors, new brain cells may be stimulated by

relearning the developmental sequences, or growth patterns, of a normal child. The human brain has progressive levels of development; each level must be sufficiently developed, in proper sequence, before proceeding to the next, and finally attaining full function. For example, a child must be able to freely move arms and legs before crawling; crawl before creeping; creep before walking.†

Frequent use of walkers and playpens can interfere with the normal sequence of brain development; these contraptions bypass the creeping and crawling stages of development by encouraging early walking. This kind of damage to brain development may be minimal, or it may seriously affect a child.

In the case of a severe injury, previously developed areas of the brain are damaged. A child must develop brain cells again in *proper sequence*. A six-year-old with brain damage must once again learn to crawl before he can walk (as did my two-year-old).

Understanding the development of the normal human brain, we can view brain-injured children in a new light. We can stop treating only symptoms — with leg braces, crutches, and operations — and work on solving the problem at its source. These are children whose brains need to *relearn* normal brain processes; they need to activate new brain cells to enable them to function at a normal, or even superior, level.

Superior nutrition, as well as high dosages of nutrients, plays an essential role in activating brain cells. Pangamic acid has been shown to stimulate speech, vitamin E to guide oxygen to the cells, niacin to increase the flow of blood to the brain, to cite a few examples. But brain-injured children need *all* nutrients to insure the entire reactivating process and ultimate health.

Our son, four years after his accident, has lived through and overcome tragic injury to his brain. The early use of superior nutrients which guide and stimulate oxygen to the cells of the brain reversed the paralysis that threatened him with severe limitations. Today Shawn is a normal, healthy, active six-year-old.

The answer for our brain-injured children lies in correct sequential patterning; superior nutrition; expanded sensory

---

†In child development terms, "crawling" is prone movement, on the stomach, with or without use of arms and legs. "Creeping" is movement on the hands and knees. For a more thorough explanation of this theory, read *What To Do about Your Brain-Injured Child,* by Glenn Doman (Doubleday, 1974).

stimulation; love and dedication. There are still unanswered questions and there are children who do not fully respond to this special treatment. But dedicated people, like those at The Institutes for the Achievement of Human Potential, are always searching for the right answers — not the conventional, ineffective ones.

The benefits of good nutrition are not limited to children with serious problems. If proper diet can help restore healthy bodies and minds to damaged children, imagine the possibilities for superior health and intelligence in normal children!

Where Do We Go from Here?

Our reactive, sensitive children are the direct result of the explosion of empty, chemical, and sugar-laden food. If toxins were introduced gradually, the human body would adjust accordingly. But they are not a gradual tide; they are a deluge. We are seeing the results in our children! Our environment is abnormal, changing so rapidly that our normal children cannot adjust.

If we refuse to feed our children the foods that destroy health, we can build health instead of disease; prevent, instead of struggling with cure.

The Ice Cream Truck Is Coming!

S tarting at the beginning of a child's life is the simplest way to have him accept nutritious food. Even so, there are always "sugar situations" that can trip you up later on. The Ice Cream Truck was the first one I faced with my son.

I had carefully avoided pointing out to Shawn that the truck with the music playing contained ice cream. But, by the time he was two, he *knew*!

Shawn was playing with his cousins in the park one quiet afternoon when we heard that familiar, tinkly music. Every kid in the park ran to greet the ice cream man, and Shawn followed. As he watched them make their purchases, I was torn. Was it fair to make my child suffer by not being included in something that all the other children were enjoying? Yet I knew that giving in just once would not end here.

With a "here goes nothing" feeling, I calmly, firmly told Shawn, "This ice cream has sugar in it. We can't buy any right now, but on the way home, we'll stop and get some honey ice cream. Okay?"

To my utter amazement, my son answered with a quick, "Okay," as he ran back to the park in pursuit of his cousins.

Although I planned to stop for the ice cream I had promised, I assumed that Shawn would have forgotten the entire episode by the time we left the park a few hours later. Not so! The second we got into the car, my two-year-old piped up, "I'm ready for my ice cream now, Mommy."

In response to my child's reaction you may be thinking:

¶ "It was easy for you since you raised your child that way."
¶ "Your child is probably quite passive. Mine would scream his/her head off until we bought some ice cream."
¶ "That is too much trouble. Besides, I would want some ice cream myself, so I would have to let my child have some."

It certainly would be easier if, from the very beginning, your child was given only healthful foods, but this is not a necessary requirement. Establishing trust between you and your child is most important in your child's acceptance of new things.

There are sensitive children who cannot handle change and react with crying, screaming, hyperactivity, or whatever the child's particular reaction is. Even though you do not have a hyperactive child, your child may appear to be when under stress. (And believe me, I include my son in this group.)

We, as parents, must be willing to work on our own nutritional problems before we attempt to change our child's eating habits. It takes time, patience, and love as you learn together. You will have to help your child deal with situations that make him feel left out or different.

Your child will not pick friends by what they eat and should not ever be encouraged to do so. Sharing knowledge with others is half the fun, and a way to grow. Let your child's friends experience real food (introduced gradually, of course). Help them understand that you serve these foods because you care — and are not withholding sugary food as a disciplinary measure.

The following are "sugar situations" that you and your child may have to deal with. Several choices are given for solving each situation since each of us is unique in the way we handle problems. A solution that adequately resolves your particular situation may not appear, but as you grow and learn with your child, you will find answers together.

Situation A: The Shopping Trip

During a shopping trip in a large mall your child becomes hungry for a snack. You can:

¶ Prepare in advance and have a snack in your purse.
¶ Promise a snack when you have finished shopping.
¶ Head for a health food store. (Many malls now have them.)

¶ Find an ice cream or confection stand that carries frozen bananas dipped in chocolate. Ask for an uncoated one. (Bananas are prefrozen and usually not dipped until ordered.)

Situation B: Halloween

When ghosts and goblins are collecting and gobbling down goodies, your child is feeling left out. You can:

¶ Throw a natural Halloween party!

¶ Use candy collected as "poker chips" that can be turned in for big prizes. This solution still includes the fun of going door to door, but it can only be used for older children. While the kids are out trick or treating, you may bake cookies or make popcorn for a surprise.

¶ Get together with friends in your neighborhood and plan to offer raisins, nuts, or other nutritious treats. When the children arrive home let them separate their treats themselves — those that are nutritious and those that are not. Have a hunt for toys as an added attraction.

Situation C: At Preschool

Your preschooler's nursery school serves white crackers and Kool-Aid for snack time. You can:

¶ Speak with the director about your feelings and offer some suggestions.

¶ Offer to make snack items. (You should expect to be paid for the price of ingredients.)

¶ Help the director search for economical, healthful snacks if money is a problem.

¶ Let everyone try a turn at making nutritious snacks if you belong to a co-op nursery school. (When needed, offer recipe ideas that require no sugar or chemicals.)

¶ Remove your child from the school if you receive rejection from the director. Anyone so closed-minded is probably not interested in your child's well-being.

Situation D: On Vacation

You are in the middle of nowhere on your vacation, the kids are starving, and there is only a McDonald's in sight. You can:

¶ Pull right into McDonald's and order unseasoned hamburgers with extra lettuce, tomato, onion — and no bun. The surprised response is usually, "No bun?" "That's right." This request usually throws the entire operation into a tizzy, and it's great fun to watch the word pass along. To add spice to your order, you may even say your family is allergic to the chemicals in white bread and you would appreciate their cooperation. If you plan ahead, you can take along a loaf of whole grain bread for your hamburgers and salad. Add milk to your order to round out your meal.

Situation E: The Sucker

Your friendly neighborhood grocer hands your child a sucker. You can:

¶ Always carry nutritious candy in your purse or car to offer as a substitute in such emergencies. Nik's treats are delicious hard drops that should satisfy your child's desire for a sucker.

¶ Stress your sincere thanks to the grocer, but explain that sugar has a negative effect on your child. Hopefully, he'll understand and not offer the sucker next time.

¶ Explain to your child (out of earshot, of course) that it was a gesture of kindness, but that many people do not realize they are hurting their bodies by ingesting sugar and chemicals.

Situation F: The Movies

On a night out at the movies, what does your child do for munchies? You can:

¶ Bring a big purse and stuff it with popcorn†, nuts, dried fruit, small bottles of juice, etc. (This is frowned upon in most theaters since they make a large profit at the snack bar, but it is unlikely that anyone will notice or say anything about it to you.)

¶ Talk to the manager or owner about including trail mix, raisins, fruit, and unsweetened juices as an experiment to find out how they sell. If he agrees, pass the word around to interested friends. Be sure to inform the local health food stores, so they can let their customers know which theater offers nutritious snacks.

¶ Stick a snack in your child's pocket if you will not be going, too.

---

† Popcorn sold in theaters is covered with artificial color and flavoring.

Situation G: The Reward

Your child's teacher rewards good work or behavior with candy. (Yes, it is still done.) You can:

¶ Have a chat with the teacher and explain your feelings. Suggest that praise, special activities, or even small toys might be used as rewards instead of food.

¶ Give the teacher a supply of nutritious snacks for your child if you cannot convince the teacher to change.

Situation H: The Neighborhood Gang

The children in your neighborhood bring out goodies and offer them to your child. You can:

¶ Supply your child with enough nuts, seeds, or fruit to share with others. (I once watched six children gather around my son, gobbling down the whole, raw almonds he was sharing. I feel certain that none of the children had ever eaten an almond in the raw before, but they went for the wholesome treat like bees to honey. And my son enjoyed the popularity.)

¶ Invite a few of your child's friends in for an afternoon of baking cookies — natural style. Rolled cookies that can be pressed into shapes usually work best. Children will usually eat anything they have made themselves.

¶ Help your child learn to refuse junk food politely. My son developed his own technique at two-and-a-half. He would ask, "Does that have sugar in it?" If the answer was yes, he would reply, "Oh, well, I don't want it." With a little coaching, it soon became, "Thank you, but I don't eat sugar."

Situation I: Relatives

Relatives sneak in sugar when your child is left in their care. You can:

¶ Take them on shopping trips to the health food store to acquaint them with a natural way of eating. You might buy lunch if the store has a restaurant or snack bar.

¶ Always supply snacks for your child to take along on visits.

¶ Supply natural ingredients for an afternoon of baking with Grandma or Auntie.

¶ Gradually ease your relatives into understanding your nutritional stand. Start with any health problem they may have; this will capture their interest.

¶ Rely on your children. As they grow aware of what foods build health, they will help your relatives understand.

Situation J: Birthday Parties

Your child is invited to a birthday party at which the usual surgary fare will be served. You can:

¶ Offer to make or buy the cake if it's a close friend.

¶ Offer to make homemade ice cream for the party. The kids can take turns with the turning of the handle or, if the machine is electric, help mix the ingredients. This will take away much of the interest in the cake.

¶ Bring a small natural cake so there are two kinds to choose from. There may be other mothers who care very much about what their children ingest but don't know how to handle the situation. (Be sure to talk this over with the birthday child's mother before bringing the cake.)

Situation K: Scout Meetings

The organization your child belongs to (Scouts, 4-H, etc.) always includes a sugary snack at their meetings. You can:

¶ Give your child a snack to take along.

¶ Give a talk on nutrition and bring some samples.

¶ Donate snacks.

¶ Talk to the other mothers about the situation and find a solution.

¶ Talk to the leader and spark some interest in him or her.

Situation L: Out of Town

You are visiting a new town and you would like to find a restaurant that serves nutritious food. You can:

¶ Look through the telephone directory under health foods.

¶ Call a health food store and ask for suggestions.

Situation M: The School Cafeteria

The school cafeteria offers a wide variety of denatured foods. You can:

¶ Pack a lunch for your child.

¶ Have your child come home for lunch.

¶ Volunteer your help to the school cafeteria.

¶ Do some research on how other schools† have successfully incorporated nutritious food into the school lunch program and present it to the school board.

---

† Write to: NUTRA, Sara Sloan, P.O. Box 13825, Atlanta, Georgia 30324
For complete and successfully applied instructions on how to incorporate natural foods into your child's lunch program in a public school situation.

¶ Organize other interested mothers to make nutritious lunches if the school won't offer them. Enter the lunchroom together to serve the lunch to your children.

Situation N: At a Friend's House

Your child is invited to a friend's home for dinner. You can:

¶ Hope for the best. A child who is well-established in nutritious foods (yours!) will know which foods to eat.

¶ Suggest simple foods for dinner if the child's mother knows and understands your feelings about nutrition. This works *only* if you are asked. Basic foods that are not mixed with sauces or in casseroles are the easiest to make. Suggest a protein (chicken, steak, or fish), vegetables (carrots, potatoes, broccoli), and possibly rice. Fruit makes a quick dessert.

¶ Invite your child's friends over frequently so they will become acquainted with a different way of eating. Serve foods that taste especially good so that the child's parents will hear about the special food at your house.

Situation O: The Candy Aisle

Your child throws a fit in the middle of the grocery store because you won't buy candy. You can:

¶ Keep in mind that your child may be reacting strongly because of an addiction to sugar. Or if you have used sugar as a reward, your denial is viewed as an undeserved punishment.

¶ Pick your child up from the floor (if having a tantrum), and gently carry your upset child from the store, staying calm and quiet yourself. This is not a punishment, but removal from a situation the child is not able to handle. Wait for your child to calm down. Then talk about what your child is feeling, and about how you feel, without anger or accusations. The situation is not resolved until you are both able to talk about it.

¶ Keep snacks in your purse as a distraction from sugary treats that were once acceptable. This may only work with very young children, such as toddlers, who are easily distracted.

¶ Prevent the problem from arising. Tell your child before you enter the grocery store that you will not be purchasing any candy in this store. You will either make some at home together or purchase a snack at the health food store after you are finished at the grocery. Better still, purchase the healthful snack beforehand if you have time.

¶ Avoid taking your child shopping with you until the craving for sugar dies down a bit.

Situation P: Teasing

Children at school tease your child about not eating junk food or about what you pack for school lunch. You can:

¶ Let your child work it out. Some children can handle difficult situations with ease; others suffer deeply from teasing. Be alert to your child's feelings, and, when it's needed, help.

¶ Invite the ringleader(s) to your home for natural cookies and milk after school. Involve the kids in a discussion of the problem, what their feelings are and why. If the ringleader(s) refuses the invitation, you may wish to visit school during lunch hour to talk with the child or children involved. (Discuss the problem with the teacher first.)

¶ Talk to your child's teacher and try to resolve the situation together. One solution might be a lesson in nutrition. The teacher might like to have you guest lecture. The children may be more accepting if you explain what natural food is all about. Be sure to bring samples of food for the children to try!

Situation Q: The Sneaky Eater

Your older child gobbles down junk food when no one else is around. You can:

¶ Be patient! It takes a long time to relearn how to eat.

¶ Supply lots of homemade cookies and candy. Stock up on favorite natural foods. Try new things!

¶ Talk about it. Explain there is no need to be sneaky — most people (yourself included) go through the same ups and downs with food.

Situation R: The Babysitter

Your child is left with a babysitter all day who stuffs your child full of white bread, Kool-Aid, and sugar goodies. You can:

¶ Change babysitters.

¶ Work out something so your child will have more nutritious food. I solved this problem by supplying food items such as natural hot dogs, honey graham crackers, yogurt, natural ice cream novelties, seeds, homemade goodies, etc. for my own child, as well as for the other children. My sitter soon supplied unsweetened apple juice, raisins, whole grain bread, fresh fruits and vegetables, ground beef, natural peanut butter, honey, etc.

¶ Talk to the mothers of the other children your sitter cares for. See if it's possible to share in the purchasing of food. This works particularly well if some of the children are hyperactive or have a specific health problem.

Situation S: Hurt Feelings

Your child refuses a homemade sugar goodie and hurts someone's feelings without meaning to. You can:

¶ Help your child be prepared. Together, work out a polite refusal to use in a difficult situation. Your child can say something like, "Thank you very much, but I am sensitive to sugar. My reactions to food sweetened with sugar are sometimes difficult for me to manage." Usually people feel uncomfortable when they cannot offer something. Have your child suggest fruits or vegetables. Juice is not a safe suggestion since often it turns out to be an artifically flavored fruit drink.

¶ Let your child handle it. There are situations that are almost impossible to get out of. If you are not with your child, it is difficult for you to understand just how hard it can be. Maybe on the next visit your child can take a cake or some cookies you have made, so the subject of natural foods can be brought up gently.

¶ Be patient with others. Help them to learn, but don't push if they are not interested. Don't make others feel guilty about their eating habits. Approach them on a level they can comfortably accept, without making them feel that their diet is hopeless.

Situation T: The Fair

At the country fair your child becomes tired and thirsty and wants a snow cone. You can:

¶ Buy a snow cone without the syrup.

¶ Come prepared with a small bottle of juice in your purse and purchase a plain snow cone. Pour the juice over it. (Or bring frozen, concentrated orange or apple juice. Let it thaw in your purse, wrapped in aluminum foil.)

Situation U: Hospitals

Your child needs to be hospitalized and the food is not suitable. You can:

¶ Ask for something more nutritious.

¶ Bring your own food. Most hospitals have a refrigerator in which you can store perishables.

¶ Ask for a food ticket for your child and go to the hospital cafeteria. There you will be able to see exactly what is being served, in what form, and choose an acceptable meal for your child.

Situation V: Selling Candy or Cookies

Your child's class or club decides to sell candy to raise funds. You can:

¶ Suggest that something other than candy be sold!

¶ Grin and bear it if it's a national organization such as the Girl Scouts. Why not donate money to the troop, without taking the cookies?

¶ Let your child decide whether or not to participate.

Situation W: Potlucks

A potluck dinner is planned and you are a bit hesitant about your family participating. You can:

¶ Bring more than one dish.

¶ Choose to eat dishes that are simple: Vegetable salad, fruit salad, chicken (taking off any coating), whole grain bread, etc. However, if you have no idea what foods others will be bringing, it is safest to bring more than one dish for your family to eat.

¶ Suggest a natural foods potluck!

¶ Have a natural potluck with Mexican, Japanese, Italian, or French food. You may taste some delicious original recipes!

Situation X: A Teenage Party at Your House

Your daughter is having her first slumber party and, of course, the food has to be just right. You want to serve nutritious food; your daughter wants to serve food that her friends will really like. You can:

¶ Go to the health food store together. Purchase chips, crackers, ice cream novelties, fruit juice sodas, a natural cake, and whatever else looks good.

¶ Make a huge bowl of fresh fruit with every fruit imaginable. (Use some frozen, unsweetened fruit if some fruits are out of season.) Serve with bowls of honey ice cream, nuts, seeds, coconut, wheat germ, and other natural toppings. Natural yogurt mixed with honey and fresh lime juice makes a delicious, refreshing fruit salad topping.

¶ Let the girls do some baking — if you can handle it! Not advisable if there are more than six at the party.

¶ Make foods that everyone likes with a natural touch — pizza*, popcorn, banana splits with hot Carob Syrup** and raw nuts.

Situation Y: Summer Camp

Your child is going away to camp for a month. You are concerned about what kind of food will be served. You can:

¶ Prep your child ahead of time. Discuss which foods are loaded with sugar and/or chemicals.

¶ Purchase your child's favorite snacks and ask the camp store to put them out for your child and others to buy. (You will have to absorb the cost to avoid complications.)

¶ Talk to the director or head cook about serving whole fruit with the dessert, so there is a choice.

¶ Choose a camp that understands nutrition and makes an effort to increase fruits and vegetables and reduce sugar foods in meal planning.

¶ Mail nutritious cookies and brownies and snacks to your child if you think it is necessary.

---

* Recipe in Chapter Thirteen.
** Recipe in Chapter Twelve

Situation Z: The Ice Cream Truck

The ice cream truck comes around the corner. You can:

¶ Ask the driver to carry some natural ice cream. Who knows, Natural Nectar [brand name] novelties could boost sales! You could even buy some ice cream novelties, give them to the driver, and then let your children "buy" them from the ice cream man.

¶ Buy an ice cream maker and interest your child in making ice cream, instead of buying the sugary variety.

¶ Offer a treat at home or a trip to get frozen yogurt.

¶ Be understanding if your child becomes upset about the ice cream truck. Remember how much fun it was to buy ice cream when you were young?

The only really good answer to this problem is to talk the ice cream man into keeping frozen yogurt or natural novelties on hand, even if you have to buy them yourself.

Dealing with Feelings

In dealing with sugar situations like these, you may feel uneasy at first about explaining your point of view to others. I have found most people very receptive when I talk to them about nutritious foods. Even so, I am still hesitant to ask others to make special preparations for my son.

When he was invited to a birthday party in an ice cream parlor, my first reaction was that he should skip it. It would be Shawn's first party without Mommy along, and I didn't think it possible for a three-year-old to face all that ice cream and cake without feeling left out or giving in. Yet, here it was again — would my son be left out of parties and outings because he could not eat what was served?

While I was mulling over this tough decision, I had a surprise visit from the birthday child's mother, whom I had only met casually a few times before. She asked if Shawn would be coming to the party. I told her honestly that I wasn't sure what to do since the party was in an ice cream parlor. (She already knew that Shawn did not eat foods containing sugar.) To her, this was not a problem — her son liked my son and wanted very much to have Shawn at his party.

Suddenly, I could see how ridiculous my fears had been. It did not matter to the friend whether Shawn ate ice cream or not;

my son mattered. The outcome was that the child's mother insisted on buying honey ice cream for Shawn. At first, I felt guilty because she had to make special preparations. But then I realized it was not my place to object — after all, she was giving the party.

Once you have embarked upon your new nutritious way of life, try to be open and honest in dealing with difficult situations. Let your child vent his feelings and have a freedom of choice.

If you child asks, "Can I have some Twinkies?", don't meet the question with, "No, that is full of sugar," Instead, ask your child to analyze the contents. You won't always be there to choose the right food and allowing your child to make decisions will strengthen self-knowledge and confidence.

Each of us must grow in our own particular way, and so must our children. If your child is resisting changes in diet, you may have reached a plateau. Give your child time to adjust to each new step. Demanding goals that your child is not quite ready to attain is just as unfair as demanding things of your child that you do not apply to yourself. Time is on your child's side, and as the body strengthens, cravings will calmly recede.

Negative Vibes

Today's world is not an easy setting for feeding your family the best possible food. A multitude of obstacles will block your progress in reshaping eating habits: television, peer pressure, high costs, common emotions and attitudes about food consumption, to name a few. Deal with these roadblocks head on and find ways to resolve them.

Television

Television may be the most serious obstacle to a healthy new way of life for your child. Television could be a fantastic vehicle for learning, but instead our children are exposed to a make-believe land laden with chemicals and sugar.

My son sits with his eyes glued to these outrageous commercials, enthralled by children dancing, singing, and having fun with their sugar goodies. He will announce, "Mommy, that has sugar in it," and then sing happily along with the ditties.

The message is quite clear — it's *fun* to eat and drink sugar! So let's all join in! (Pop some fluoride pills and don't worry about cavities.) Daily brainwashing by sugar commercials will eventually take hold.

Protecting our children from television is not always easy. Most of us are well aware of the effect television has on our children, yet it buys us quiet moments to ourselves. We parents need time to pull ourselves together; finding ways other than TV to occupy children is time-consuming and not always successful.

Older children are capable of understanding that you need

quiet moments to yourself, but it is usually impossible to keep young ones occupied by themselves for very long. One alternative to sticking your child in front of the television set is a mothers' play group. Gather a few friends who have children in the same age range as your own and pick two or three mornings a week to trade children. If you have a large group of children you may need two mothers to supervise.

This rotation of children can also be applied to babysitting. You'll have fewer worries about the care your children receive because of the reciprocal arrangement — "You take care of mine and I'll take care of yours."

There will still be times when you just want a moment to yourself without having to call a friend to watch your children. Keep on hand special toys like bubbles, paint, Playdoh, dishes for a tea party, anything your child particularly enjoys. Put on records or tapes of interest to your child, for your child to listen to while playing alone.

Occasional viewing of educational programs is a fun way to learn, but watch with your child. If necessary, do ironing or sewing at the same time. Sesame Street has become a sharing experience for our family — my husband, Shawn and I talk and laugh together while Bert and Ernie entertain us.

Relatives

In raising children, we have all faced some interference from relatives. Grandma means well, but she is of the old school when it comes to nutrition. She may believe that part of being a grandmother is making sugar-laden goodies for grandchildren. Since she sees denial of sugar as a punishment, she may take quite a stand on her right to give her grandchildren sweets. All good children are rewarded with sugar, hence *goodies* got their name! Besides, aren't children missing out on one of the best things in life if they aren't allowed to eat sugar? Acceptance of new things comes slowly to many and must be dealt with patiently.

Not allowing your child to consume sugar does *not* mean your child cannot have cake, cookies, and ice cream. It simply means that the ingredients in these items are changed so that they can build health.

Using desserts for reward and denial promotes an emotional desire for sweets that is difficult to break. It connects acceptance, love and good behavior with sugar. The emotional cycle repeats itself if we pass it on to our children. Avoid rewarding your child with *any* food. A reward should be in the form of affection so that your child will know just how much you love him. Surprisingly, your children may help relatives understand your position better than you can! Children have an uncanny knack of being totally honest.

"Grandma, does that have sugar in it?" or "That will hurt my teeth," are subtle refusals that Grandma can't ignore.

Convenience

Many mothers are now learning the joy of freedom in being their own person. In reaching out to find ourselves, we must find the delicate balance between time for ourselves and time for our children. Our children's nutritional needs often get lost in the shuffle when we choose convenient fast foods over time in the kitchen.

To pop a frozen dinner into the oven, to open a can, to add water to a cake mix, to mix up Jello from a package, to use pre-whipped cream is so easy — but is it worth it? Convenience foods are advertised as tasting like homemade or even better than homemade, yet it seems a bit ridiculous to me to choose artificial food over the real thing. I want 100 percent real food for my family because I want 100 percent health for them.

As food awareness grows, so does the availability and variety of nutritious food. There are lots of natural convenience foods — cake mixes, macaroni and cheese, pizza, burger mixes, frozen waffles, canned and dry soup mix — but, just like artificial fast foods, you pay for the convenience. Try new products, but save money by organizing your kitchen. Keeping staples on hand and doing a little advance preparation can offer you quick escape from the kitchen.

Time-saving Ideas

¶ Gelatin can be prepared in exactly the same amount of time as Jello! Just keep unflavored gelatin on hand and use your favorite juice.

¶ Try making your own TV dinners. Freeze leftovers in individual trays. For example, if you serve meatloaf and zucchini for dinner, fill sections of the tray with meatloaf, zucchini, and possibly applesauce. Health Valley [brand name] makes natural frozen dinners. Remember to add a big salad when serving this sort of meal!

53

¶ Make a large amount of salad and put it in an airtight container (undressed). When someone in the family is left to fend for food alone, there is a salad ready to eat.

¶ Whenever you bake, make double the amount. Freeze individual portions for lunchboxes or snacks.

¶ Pre-grind seeds (such as sunflower and sesame) and store in the refrigerator.

¶ Keep a well-stocked pantry. Label everything in bold letters. Use large jars so you will not have to keep filling them.

¶ Freeze soup in portions small enough for one person, as well as in portions large enough for a family meal.

¶ Use one refrigerator shelf for snacks. Have fresh fruit, cut-up vegetables, Yogurt Dip*, muffins*, cheese, or any of your child's favorite foods. This shelf offers your child a smorgasbord and saves you the trouble of jumping up and down preparing snacks.

Meals do not have to be complicated to be nutritious. An omelet and a large salad is quick and much more nutritious than any of the fast foods you could buy.

Many convenience appliances are now on the market — super blenders, food processors, juicers, slowcookers, dehydrators, and other special cookware. Choose a good blender first. As your finances permit, you might invest in a Champion Juicer, a three-tiered sprouter, a seed grinder, a vegetable steamer, and a crockpot. The effects of microwaves are unknown. Until it has been proven that there is no danger in using microwave ovens, I would avoid them.

Expense

Many families feel that eating natural food is too expensive. I feel it is a simple matter of priorities. Real juice does cost more than artificially colored and flavored sugar water, but there is no comparison. The media would like you to believe that the only nutrient in real juice is vitamin C, so why not save money by buying a mixture of sugar, color, flavor, water, and a bit of vitamin C? It is much cheaper to give your child a vitamin C tablet.

The addition of a few B vitamins to sugar cereals or sugary baked goods is also a meaningless gesture. Those B vitamins are used up when the body metabolizes the sugar in the product.

---

* Recipes in Chapter Thirteen.

Your child's body will probably use every bit of vitamin C added to an artificial drink just to detoxify the chemicals in the same drink.

Natural food co-ops are gaining in popularity as more families care about the foods they eat and as the price of all food soars. You may wish to start your own co-op or join an existing one to help you deal with high food costs. Unfortunately, the unappealing appearance of some badly-run co-ops has earned co-ops a reputation as being counterculture stores and they fail to attract the average shopper. Remember there *are* well-run, clean, attractive co-ops. If you aren't satisfied with co-ops in your area, start your own.

Growing your own fruits and vegetables can be fun, but, if you aren't interested in gardening, visit a farmers' market instead. When buying at the grocery store, remember many fruits and vegetables are waxed, oiled, or dyed to prolong shelf life. The mineral oil on cucumbers and other produce, when ingested, carries off the body's fat-soluble vitamins A, D, E and K.

The Real Thing

As in any industry there are always those whose only motive is profit. Products by a few companies give the entire health food industry a bad name. Any product that contains white flour, sugar, or any questionable additive is not a natural food and should not be labeled as such. In buying the most nutritious food for your family you need to read *all* labels. Don't take it for granted that if you buy something in a health food store it has to be good for you.

There are a few excellent companies that can be trusted to use the very best ingredients in their products:

Arrowhead Mills	Lifestream
Better Way	Manna Mixins
Bronner	Pure and Simple
Chico-San	Schiff
De Sousa	Shiloh Farms
Desert Gold	Sonoma
Elf Liberty	Sovex
Erewhon	Walnut Acres
Health Valley	Westbrae

Other companies produce some very good products, but do include in their line products containing sugar and/or white flour, so *check the labels:*

Barbara's Bakery	Hain
De Bole	Lakewood Juices
Elams	Soken
El Molino Mills	Stone-Burr
Fearn	Natural Nector

The Power of the Grocery Store

You cannot buy all the nutritious food you need in a grocery store. But as demand for nutritious foods grows, so do health food departments in grocery stores. You probably purchase your dairy products, meat, fish, and produce at the grocery store. As you learn more, you may want to search out food grown without chemicals.

Acceptable foods can be found in the supermarket:

Freezer — Unsweetened whole frozen fruit, concentrated orange and apple juice, frozen vegetables in plastic bags or boxes (not mixed with sauces), fish (not breaded), Jones and Rich's sausage.

Canned Foods — Water-packed tuna, unsweetened apple-sauce, pineapple packed in its own juice, Dole peaches, pears, and apricots packed in natural fruit juice, unsweetened juices such as pineapple, grape, apple. Martinelli's sparkling cider is good for special occasions.

Dairy — Plain yogurt, acidophilus milk, eggs, natural cheeses (only those without coloring), butter (without coloring), buttermilk, and regular milk.

Produce — Any fresh fruit or vegetables available. Watch out for the mineral oil on cucumbers, wax on apples, and dye on oranges.

Staples — Unflavored gelatin (Knox [brand name]), beans, whole grains, whole wheat flour, honey, raisins, natural peanut butter.

Breads and Cereals — Check labels carefully. You may come across some breads and cereals made with whole grains and sweetened with only honey or raisin syrup.

Seasonings and condiments — Hollywood [brand name] mayonnaise, oil, and dressing. You may find dressing under other labels that are natural. It is possible to find pure mustard, but ketchup always contains sugar. Herbs and spices are usually alright, but do not buy any mixed seasonings such as gravy mix or spaghetti seasoning. These are usually full of chemicals. *Cookies and Crackers* — It is doubtful you will find any cookies without sugar. If you do, they will be located in the health food section. Crackers with whole grain flour are a little easier to find, but choice is limited. Look for Akmak [brand name] crackers as a good substitute for saltines. *Meats* — Only fresh meat, turkey, chicken, and fish.

I cannot obtain all the foods I need in a grocery store. So many foods contain objectionable ingredients that I become frustrated reading labels. You too may find your trips to the grocery store less frequent as you read more labels!

The Time To Be Jolly

Holidays traditionally mean an explosion of goodies. Quantities of denatured food are literally thrust upon a child during holidays. The child's ability to cope will largely depend on how parents handle the situation.

No child should ever feel denied a pleasure that all other children experience. A child *raised* with natural foods will not have as difficult an emotional adjustment to make as the child who has learned to equate sugar with happiness and love. Nevertheless, everyone has weak moments when they gobble down an unspeakable sugar goodie. Providing holiday foods that are new and exciting, as well as nutritious, will eliminate impulsive attacks of sugar ingestion. If and when your child experiences a setback, handle it lightly. This is part of the learning process. Talk about your own problems in learning to eat nutritious food and help your child accept mistakes as growth, without guilt.

Valentine's Day

This day for sweetness and expression of love need not be celebrated with sugar. A tradition in our family is to exchange gifts. Include cookies and cake in the shape of hearts if your family desires.

Your child's class at school will probably exchange valentines at a party with refreshments, so send an alternative to the usual sugar cookies and candy. If there are other mothers interested in nutritious refreshments, get together to plan and make some treats.

Red Party Punch: Mix Health Valley strawberry nectar or R.W. Knudsen and Sons Cranberry Nector with naturally carbonated mineral water.

Valentine Hearts: Use any rolled cookie recipe that uses only natural ingredients (see recipe section of this book or use any of your own favorite recipes). Press into shape of hearts. Ice with Cream Cheese Frosting* colored pink with beet juice or Earth Grown natural food coloring.

Party Favors Plus: Carob-covered nuts (*only* those that are unsweetened), fruit kabobs (use fresh pineapple and whole frozen strawberries or bing cherries), Strawberry Fruit Leather*, popcorn balls.

Easter

Most children find chocolate bunnies, marshmallow chicks, egg-shaped candies, jelly beans, and artifically colored boiled eggs on Easter morning. It doesn't have to be this way! Your child can have basket things as delightful or more so than a pile of sugary goodies.

Natural Easter Eggs: Boil a dozen eggs with two tablespoons of vinegar for 15 minutes so natural dyes will take easily.

Red — Beet juice. Cook beets, blend and strain. Or juice raw beets in a juicer.

Blue — Cabbage. Chop 1 cup red cabbage, steep like tea with 1 tps. vinegar until water turns desired shade; strain.

Yellow — Saffron. Steep about 2 T. saffron in 1 cup boiling water; strain.

Orange — Onion skins. Boil ½ cup onion skin with 1½ cups of water for five minutes, steep, and strain.

Softened wax (not melted) may be applied to the eggs with a pin or paint brush to produce designs.

Soak eggs until they become the desired shade. For different colors, dip dried, colored eggs into another color.

Remove wax by melting near a candle.

The Natural Easter Basket: Fill with toys, fruit, carob-covered nuts or raisins (only unsweetened), Burry's carob bunnies, honey taffy, or any other natural candy your child enjoys. Fill plastic eggs with nuts, seeds, dried fruit, money, and homemade Marshmallows*.

---

* Recipe in Chapter Thirteen

Birthdays

A natural birthday party does not require any more prepara
tion than a sugary one. If there is not a natural bakery in your
city, make your own cake. Hold it! No excuses about making a
cake from scratch — you can use a packaged mix from Elf
Liberty [brand name] if you are worried about a homemade
cake not turning out right.

Make Butter Frosting*, adding carob powder, banana,
coconut, lemon, or peanut butter, etc. for flavoring and color.
Make contrasting colors for writing on the cake by adding to the
frosting beet juice for pink, carrot juice for orange, grape juice
for lavender, chlorophyll for green, and other natural colors†
derived from fruits and vegetables. Garnish the cake with fresh
flowers, nuts, seeds, or raisins.

Serve honey ice cream, frozen yogurt (check ingredients for
purity), or make your own while the party is in progress. Fill a
pinata with small toys and wrapped honey candy from the
health food store.

If you plan a meal for the party, make foods that are easy to
eat. Crunchy Chicken*, tacos, or homemade Pizza A La
Natural* are usually a hit.

The Cake: Make cake from a natural mix, buy the cake at a
natural bakery, or make your own from a recipe in this book.
For guests younger than five, cupcakes are easier to handle —
and easier for you to clean up.

Drinks: Fruit juice with naturally carbonated mineral water
will go over well. Make root beer floats with Health Valley root
beer and honey ice cream or orange juice floats with fresh
orange juice and natural strawberry ice cream.

Ice Cream: Frozen yogurt or honey ice cream is great by
itself. Or let kids make their own sundaes and banana splits. Set
out dishes of Carob Syrup**, Caramel Syrup**, homemade
Marshmallows*, cut-up fruit (fresh or frozen berries, crushed
pineapple), nuts, raisins, seeds, coconut, real maple syrup, carob

---

* Recipe in Chapter Thirteen.

** Recipes in Chapter Twelve. See "Caramel Apples" for Caramel Syrup
recipe.

† Convenient natural colors are available in orange, green, red, and yellow
from Earth Grown (manufactured by Sorbee Sugarless International)

chips (unsweetened), honey granola, or chopped dates. Top with whipped cream (sweetened with honey) and bing cherries (fresh or frozen). Natural ice cream is also available in cups, in a mold, or as novelties. Natural Nector [brand name] honey ice cream novelties are outrageously good.

Favors: Keep favors light. Nuts, seeds, and dried fruit in cups should keep children busy while waiting to be served.

Halloween

A party is a good way to corral the stampede for candy at Halloween. Several interested parents may want to get together to give a party for their little ghouls.

Spooky stories, carving pumpkins, bobbing for apples, a spook house, puppet show, a hunt for hidden spiders could be more fun than trick-or-treating. Let your child choose the entertainment — children know what would be the most fun for them.

You will probably want to center refreshments around apples and pumpkins.

Witch's Brew: Orange juice with Perrier [brand name], hot apple cider with cinnamon sticks, or Martinelli's [brand name] sparkling apple cider. Serve drinks in hollowed-out apples.

Goblin Gobbles: Gingerbread*, Pumpkin Pie*, Caramel Apples,** Apple Crisp*. Roasted pumpkin seeds are yummy!

Christmas

The season to be jolly is also the season to eat, eat, eat! If you get baking mania around Christmas, like I do, put it to good use! Try out new recipes or experiment with whole food substitutions in your favorite recipes. Your wholesome baked goods make ideal presents for friends and family.

Parties, visiting, and traveling present the kinds of adjustments discussed in Chapter Six. The worst situation of all is the visit to Santa. When the lovable, old fellow places candy in the hands of our children, we have to figure out *how to get the candy out of the child's hand!* The best solution is to not let it get there in the first place. To accomplish this you can:

* Recipes in Chapter Thirteen
** Recipe in Chapter Twelve

¶ Call ahead to find out what Santa is handing out. Sometimes coloring books are offered instead of candy. Don't take any chances, though, since most Santas do hand out candy.

¶ Go with another adult who will keep your child busy in the toy department. Meanwhile, you can provide Santa with something acceptable to give your child (such as a Burry's [brand name] carob Santa or a small toy).

¶ Ask Santa's helper to give Santa the word about no candy.

Jolly Moments

Holidays are to be enjoyed. By making them natural, as well as fun, you are showing your child that natural is not dull. Natural foods can have great appeal to children and can be joyfully accepted!

To Be or Not To Be
(a Veggy)

Vegetarianism was once thought to be a diet for eccentrics — those who swilled carrot juice and munched on alfalfa sprouts, soy burgers, and wheat germ. It is impractical and extreme for most of us to try to exist on such a diet . . . but not any more so than eating meat and potatoes exclusively.

The average American diet consists mostly of overcooked proteins and starches. Raw foods are almost entirely absent from the typical diet. An occasional salad of iceberg lettuce, tomatoes, and croutons, and a piece of fruit now and then are usually the only raw foods ever eaten.

Some foods must be cooked to release certain vitamins. The vitamin A (carotene) in carrots, for example, is more readily available if the carrots have been cooked to break down the fibrous cellulose. Carrots have more to offer than Vitamin A, however. All raw foods contain not only essential vitamins and minerals, but enzymes.

Enzymes are vital in breaking down foods into substances the body can utilize and in building new, living cells. In fact, without enzymes, no life would be possible. Scientists think this is why fevers over 108 degrees are fatal: the life-sustaining enzymes are killed by high temperatures.

Enzymes in foods are similarly destroyed by high temperatures in cooking. Enzymes naturally present in raw food work in conjunction with corresponding enzymes already present in the body. Together they make digestion possible. If food enzymes are destroyed by cooking, the body must produce more enzymes. Consequently, food cannot be properly broken down.

The poorly assimilated particles become irritants to the body's system: allergic reactions result (see Chapter Five). Our children's allergies will continue as long as they lack proper enzymes for digestion, absorption, and growth. Overcooked foods destroy enzymes; raw foods provide them.

Children especially benefit from eating raw foods, instead of denatured ones, because of their growing bodies and minds. Vegetarianism is unnecessarily drastic, but getting raw foods into a child is essential. It can also be difficult. Set a beautiful bowl of salad before some children (and even some adults) and they will complain,

"I don't eat grass."

We must adjust our diets to the tastes and needs of our family.

Getting Children to Eat the Impossible

Juicing fruits and vegetables is a delicious and concentrated way to get raw food into your child (and yourself, too). Most children like fruit juices. Add a *small* amount of vegetable juice to fruit juices, gradually increasing the amount over a period of time, and the combination will supply vitamins, minerals, and enzymes. The purchase of a juicer would be a worthwhile investment. If a juicer is a luxury you cannot afford, a blender and a little creativity can whip up some healthful concoctions, too.

Let your child experiment with combinations of juices and discover what tastes best. *Never* leave any child alone with a juicer or blender, though.

Blender Drinks

MINT TINGLE

fresh pineapple juice
very small quantity of celery,
    parsley, and spinach
mint to taste

ROSEY RED

fresh tomato juice
fresh beet juice (small amount)
bit of lemon

APPLE ZAZZLE

---

fresh apple juice
handful of alfalfa sprouts
fresh papaya juice

ORANGEY ORANGE

---

fresh orange juice
fresh carrot juice (start with 1 T. and work up)

Snacks

Keep a tray of cut-up vegetables with dip at all times in your refrigerator. Children love to dip so much that they might not notice what they are eating with the dip. Watch out for cheaters — sometimes the little rascals will lick the dip from veggies and discard them like toothpicks.

*Dips**
cottage cheese and chives
peanut butter
mashed avocado and lemon juice
yogurt with Hain [brand name] onion soup mix

Veggies

turnips	celery
beets	cucumber
broccoli	green pepper
carrots	tomato
cauliflower	zucchini

The vegetable or fruit sandwich (the Un-Sandwich, Chapter Two) is also a handy offering for a child of any age. Some fruits and vegetables have a built-in space for fillings, others may be sliced and used like the "bread" of the sandwich. Try some of these:

¶ Celery stuffed with nut butters or cheese
¶ Cored apple stuffed with a slice of cheese or a cheese spread*
¶ Cucumber boats filled with tuna or egg salad
¶ Avocado halves with shrimp and cheese mixture

---

* Recipes in Chapter Thirteen.

Side dishes at mealtime need not be overcooked vegetables in heavy sauces. Cut up and store fruit salad in your refrigerator, so it is always ready. Use as a topping for yogurt, a light snack by itself, or as a quick dessert. Finely grated vegetable salads like coleslaw and Carrot-Raisin* keep well, and can be used for lunch or dinner.

Children love watching things grow. Sprouting seeds and grains in a sprouter or a mason jar is a simple, fun way to obtain raw food. A three-tiered sprouter that grows three types of sprouts at once is made by Biosnacky. Keep it on your table for convenient nibbling — it's also quite a conversation piece.

A bowl of fruit supplies a fast snack for your child to grab on the way out to play. Vary apples, pears, bananas, oranges with whatever other fruits are in season. Toddlers love bite-size berries. How ironic it is that many American families use a bowl of *plastic* fruit as a *decoration* for their tables!

Food Rhythm

Vegetarians are often lumped in one class — people who do not eat meat. But there are many kinds of vegetarians. There are those who:

¶ Exclude only red meat from their diet.
¶ Exclude only red meat and fowl.
¶ Exclude red meat, fowl, fish.
¶ Exclude red meat, fowl, fish, eggs.
¶ Exclude red meat, fowl, fish, eggs, milk products.

Some vegetarian diets stress grains while others lean more toward fruits and/or vegetables. Some vegetarians care little about the quantities of sugar and chemicals they ingest as long as they don't consume any animal products. Others eat only the purest of food. Being a vegetarian does not necessarily mean one is in the best of health. Many prepared vegetarian foods contain chemicals and sugar.

Some vegetarians enjoy excellent health on a diet that excludes all animal products, but they are a very small group. Even those who consume milk products are often unable to remain healthy. Sadly, too many vegetarians have a dull, hollow look in their eyes and a droop to their shoulders that says their diet is completely out of balance.

---

* Recipe in Chapter Thirteen.

Vegetarians must carefully balance their diet with food they are able to assimilate properly. For example, hypoglycemics are frequently unable to break down starchy grains and beans, and would do better stressing raw fruits and vegetables, seeds, nuts, and nutritional yeast.

If you choose a vegetarian diet for your child, watch closely to see if the diet really fulfills the child's needs. Does your child *look* healthy, is he/she ever sick, and is he/she energetic (but not hyperactive)? A vegetarian diet for your family should include high quality protein foods such as nutritional yeast, eggs, nuts, seeds, milk products, sprouts, avocado, and occasionally fish and fowl (include organs) to insure an ultimate level of health.

Vit-A-Man!

H ow do you determine which children's chewable vitamins will benefit your child the most? Is it the shape or flavor, the advertisement, your child's preference, the content of iron, or the doctor's recommendation? Making the right choice is not easy since most of us really don't know what we're looking for.

There are some experts who claim that vitamin supplements are unnecessary, or that a minimal dosage of a select few will bring about glowing health. The limited potencies available for children are so unbalanced that, looking at the analysis, you would conclude iron is the only necessary mineral, the B vitamins are a family of only seven, and that vitamin E is nonexistent.

ANALYSIS OF VITAMINS FOR CHILDREN

	Sample 1	Sample 2	Sample 3
Vitamin A	3500 I.U.	2500 I.U.	3500 I.U.
Vitamin D	400 I.U.	400 I.U.	400 I.U.
Vitamin C	40 mg.	60 mg.	60 mg.
Vitamin E	none	15 I.U.	none
Thiamine (B_1)	1.1 mg.	1.05 mg.	.8 mg.
Riboflavin (B_2)	1.2 mg.	1.2 mg.	1.3 mg.
Pyroxidine (B_6)	1.2 mg.	1.05 mg.	1 mg.
Cobalamin (B_{12})	5 mcg.	4.5 mcg.	2.5 mcg.
Niacin (B_3)	15 mg.	13.5 mg.	14 mg.
Pantothenic Acid (B_5)	5 mg.	none	5 mg.
Folic Acid	.1 mg.	.15 mg.	.25 mg.
Iron	10 mg.	15 mg.	12 mg.

The base of these formulas is not always listed. Sometimes only the words "natural sweeteners, artificial colors, and artificial flavors" appear on the label. By reading the ingredients of similar preparations, it becomes clear that the "natural" sweetener is sugar (sucrose).

Typical Vitamin Base — Sucrose, steric acid, dextrin, gelatin, artificial color, artificial flavor, glycerides of steric, and palmitic acids.

Establishing a Balance

The nutritional needs of children are intricate. Vitamins and minerals work together, and must be supplied in adequate, balanced amounts to insure ultimate health. Iron is essential, but not more so than any other mineral. Stressing the importance of a single mineral leads us to believe that other minerals are adequately supplied by a normal diet.

All the vitamins and minerals a child requires could not be put into one tablet — it would be too large to swallow. Supplementing your child's diet with chewable tablets or liquid drops (for your very little ones) is helpful, but not the complete answer to preventing deficiencies. Concentrated foods which contain large quantities of vitamins and minerals in a natural balance are needed.

Choosing Sources of Nutrients

When choosing a tablet or liquid supplement for your child, select one which:

¶ Offers a high, balanced dosage.
¶ Contains no sugar or chemicals.
¶ Your child will accept.

Children frequently reject chewable supplements because of the strong taste of B vitamins. After you carefully check ingredients, it would be a good idea to have your child taste the supplement. A one-daily supplement will be far from perfect so you may do better purchasing chewable vitamins separately:

¶ Vitamin A and D (combined) — 5000 I.U. and 400 I.U.
¶ Vitamin E — 100 to 200 I.U.
¶ Vitamin C — 250 to 500 I.U.

Add a mineral-balanced nutritional yeast to your child's diet to supply the B vitamins and minerals.

Vitamin-mineral chewables should be sweetened with fructose instead of sucrose (table sugar). Nature's Plus [brand name] offers a good-tasting and well-balanced chewable mineral supplement: Mini Mins with chelated minerals. (Chelated minerals are those in which the minerals are bonded onto amino acids to aid in assimilation.) Richlife [brand name] has available chewable Mighty Mouse vitamins which are often quite appealing to young children. It is still important to use nutritional yeast as a supplement, along with these chewable vitamins and minerals, to meet requirements for *all* the B vitamins — those that have been isolated and those that have not.

The nutritional needs of nursing infants may be met with liquid vitamin C and A-D-E drops (or cod liver oil and wheat germ oil). The B vitamins and minerals will be in breast milk, if the mother adheres to an excellent diet, heavily spiked with nutritional yeast. As the infant begins to eat food, add nutritional yeast to the child's diet to supply additional nutrients.

No nutrient acts independently of another. Carbohydrates, fats, protein, vitamins, minerals, and water are essential to life, but quantities necessary to maintain ultimate health vary according to heredity, age, sex, size, environment, and activity. Because each of us is unique, it is difficult to give exact requirements for a specific nutrient. But if you provide a variety of superior foods along with supplements, you can feel comfortable your child is getting necessary nutrients.

How Vitamins Help Our Children

Vitamin A is a fat-soluble vitamin that builds resistance against infections, prevents eye diseases, aids in the digestion of protein, nourishes skin and hair, and builds strong bones and teeth. Vitamin A should be taken with vitamin D, vitamin E, and a source of fat to insure its absorption.

Deficiencies may cause patches of dry scaly skin, night blindness, soft tooth enamel, and decreased resistance to infection. In severe deficiencies, damage may occur to the central nervous system, because the brain and other parts of the central nervous system continue to grow without a corresponding increase in the size of the bony structures.

Sources: Fish liver oils, dark-colored fruits and vegetables (carrots, yams, melon, tomato, apricots, etc.), eggs, and whole milk.

The B Vitamins are a water-soluble complex that function closely together. A specific balance among the B group is necessary for the interrelated function of each member. Since all of the B vitamins have not been isolated, it is important to eat foods containing high amounts of the B complex. Supplements containing only one (or a few) of the B vitamins create deficiencies by increasing the need for the neglected ones. When enough friendly bacteria are present, the body will produce some of its own B vitamins. Friendly bacteria are destroyed by antibiotics. If your child must take an antibiotic, re-establish friendly bacteria with yogurt or liquid acidophilus culture.

The B complex is necessary for the metabolism of carbohydrates, fat, and protein. The metabolism of refined sugar uses up B vitamins at a terrific rate, wasting this complex of vitamins essential to the digestive system, the blood, the brain and nervous system.

Thiamine (B_1) promotes growth, stimulates brain action (learning capacity), stabilizes the appetite, maintains a healthy nervous system, helps in the metabolism of carbohydrates, and prevents nausea caused by air or sea sickness.

Sources: Nutritional yeast, organ meats, blackstrap molasses, egg yolk, soybeans, nuts, seeds, milk, wheat germ.

Riboflavin (B_2) is necessary for healthy eyes, skin, nails, and hair. It prevents eyes from being bloodshot, sensitive (to light), or burning. Other symptoms of deficiency are cracks and sores at the corners of the mouth; scaly skin around the nose/mouth/forehead/ears; and dull or oily hair. After ingestion of high potency B vitamins, urine will be a rich yellow color due to excretion of excess riboflavin. This harmless reaction is a sign that the body is well-saturated with B vitamins.

Sources: Milk products, nutritional yeast, almonds, sunflower seeds, organ meats, and wheat germ.

Pyridoxine (B_6) is beneficial to allergies, hypoglycemia, and convulsions caused by a B_6 and magnesium deficiency. It activates enzymes, prevents tooth decay, is a natural diuretic. Since it is necessary in the synthesis of protein, the more protein eaten, the higher the level of pyridoxine required. The production of antibodies, circulation to fingers and toes, and normal functioning of the brain and nervous system require pyridoxine.

Magnesium works closely with B_6 in controlling bedwetting. Pyridoxine is used in nutrient therapy to treat learning disabilities.

Sources: Pecans, nutritional yeast, wheat germ, blackstrap molasses, egg yolk, and green leafy vegetables.

Cobalamin (B_{12}) injections are given by many doctors because it is difficult to assimilate when taken by mouth. Cobalamin is essential in producing red blood cells and growth in children.

Sources: Organ meats, eggs, milk, nutritional yeast, sunflower seeds, and bee pollen.

Niacin improves blood circulation, thus improving concentration and increasing energy level. Optimal doses of niacin are used to treat hyperactivity, learning disabilities, and some mental disorders. Deficiencies may result in canker sores, insomnia, coated tongue, digestive upsets, irritability, diarrhea, fears, acne, fatigue, and headaches.

A large dose of niacin can make skin flush with a tingling sensation on the face, ears, and sometimes arms and legs. Supplements, or even nutritional yeast in large quantities, can cause this flushing. It is not an allergic reaction, but due to the dilation of the blood vessels, a normal reaction. If nutritional yeast is introduced slowly into the diet and eaten with other foods, this reaction will not occur. Brewers yeast flakes cause a stronger reaction than balanced yeast powder. Because the synthetic form of niacin, called niacinamide, does not produce flushing, it is used when large quantities are required.

Sources: Nutritional yeast, liver, wheat germ, sunflower seeds, milk products, seafood, and fowl.

Paba stimulates the growth of beneficial intestinal bacteria. It is essential to the formation of blood cells and for healthy skin. When applied topically as a cream, it soothes burns.

Sources: Nutritional yeast, yogurt, liver, wheat germ, blackstrap molasses, and green leafy vegetables.

Pantothenic Acid is an important stress reliever. It stimulates the adrenal glands, speeds recovery and prevents illness, and is helpful in relieving hypoglycemia, asthma, and allergies. It is frequently used in nutrient therapy for children.

Sources: Nutritional yeast, wheat germ, liver, egg yolk, blackstrap molasses, and whole grains.

Folic Acid is essential for the growth and division of all body cells, making it especially important during early pregnancy. It promotes growth, helps build antibodies, and is necessary for the formation of red blood cells.

Sources: Nutritional yeast, dark green leafy vegetables, liver, wheat germ, mushrooms, and nuts.

Choline and inositol are components of lecithin which function closely together in brain cell nutrition. Choline regulates and improves liver and gall bladder function. Inositol is essential to the health of cells in bone marrow, eye membranes, and intestines. The body will produce its own lecithin if the correct nutrients are present. The use of lecithin derived from soy has become popular as assurance against choline and inositol deficencies and to keep fats emulsified in the bloodstream.

Sources: Lecithin, nutritional yeast, and liver.

Biotin assists in the metabolism of proteins and fats. Deficiencies may cause fatigue, eczema, skin disorders, loss of appetite, and heart abnormalities.

Sources: Nutritional yeast, liver, and brown rice.

To insure the balance and ingestion of *all* the B vitamins, use nutritional yeast, liver, wheat germ, seeds, and nuts liberally in your child's diet.

Vitamin C (ascorbic acid) fights bacterial infections (especially colds and flu); reduces the effects of allergic reactions, and maintains the health of the gums, bones, and teeth. Being water-soluble, it must be replenished daily. Vitamin C detoxifies toxic chemicals and, in doing so, helps sensitive, allergic children get rid of toxins they are unable to handle. The first sign of deficiency is usually bleeding gums or bruising easily.

The **bioflavonoids** are part of the C complex. They strengthen capillary walls and prevent the destruction of vitamin C in the body by oxidation.

Sources: Citrus fruits, sprouts, green pepper, broccoli, rose hips, tomatoes, and strawberries supply vitamin C. Buckwheat, the white pulp of citrus fruits, fresh fruits and vegetables supply the bioflavonoids.

Vitamin D needs fat and vitamin A to be absorbed. Vitamin D helps build bone structure; without vitamin D the body cannot assimilate the minerals it needs. Vitamin D is also needed for normal blood clotting, and to maintain the health of the nervous system.

Sources: Fish liver oils, egg yolk, organ meats, mushrooms, and sunflower seeds.

Vitamin E has been popularly associated with sex and reproduction. Yet, the most important function of vitamin E is that it is essential to the cells' utilization of oxygen. It does prevent infertility, stillbirth, miscarriages, and menstrual disorders. But it also helps hypoglycemia, skin disorders, glandular dysfunction, muscle weakness and crossed eye muscles. It increases endurance and stamina; protects hormones and fat-soluble vitamins from being destroyed by oxygen. Applied topically, it promotes healing and lessens scarring.

Sources: Cold-pressed, unrefined oils (wheat germ oil especially), wheat germ, sprouts, nuts, seeds, grains.

Vitamin F, or unsaturated fatty acids, are essential for normal glandular activity, healthy skin-hair-mucous membranes, and in promoting growth. Cold-pressed oils are good sources of unsaturated fatty acids, but an increase in oil must be accompanied with an increase of vitamin E.

Sources: Unrefined, cold-pressed vegetable oils.

Vitamin K is necessary for normal clotting of blood and normal liver function. Friendly bacteria in the intestines will promote the growth of Vitamin K.

Sources: Kelp, alfalfa, egg yolks, green leafy vegetables, and liver.

Vitamin T is a growth-promoting vitamin that also encourages appetite.

Source: Sesame seeds.

How Minerals Help Our Children

All minerals work together as a unit, the lack of one will throw all the minerals out of balance. The need for iron and calcium is often stressed by doctors or advertising, yet other minerals are equally essential and just as difficult to obtain.

Calcium has a calming effect on the system. It speeds healing, builds and maintains bones and teeth, and regulates heart action. A balance of calcium and magnesium is almost impossible in the typical denatured American diet.

Sources: Milk, cheese, sesame seeds, almonds, sunflower seeds, green leafy vegetables, and blackstrap molasses.

Magnesium is a sorely neglected mineral that plays an important role in our energy level. It also helps form enamel on teeth, may prevent or control convulsions (with pyridoxine), and is a natural tranquilizer. Severe deficiencies affect the brain with clouded thinking, confusion, disorientation, and depression. Magnesium deficiency is often associated with bedwetting. Synthetic vitamin D, such as that used to fortify pasteurized milk, often binds magnesium and carries it out of the body.

Sources: Nuts, sunflower seeds, sesame seeds, dark green vegetables, and whole grains.

Phosphorus is necessary for efficient mental activity, kidney function, strong bones and teeth, and in carbohydrate metabolism.

Sources: Milk products, eggs, whole grains, nuts, seeds, and fish.

Potassium, Chlorine, and Sodium work together to regulate fluid on both sides of the cellular wall. The massive amounts of sodium (salt) in processed foods produce an imbalance which causes potassium to be lost in the urine. Potassium is essential for proper function of the nervous system, heart, and kidneys. Sodium and chlorine help in the production of hydrochloric acid.

Sources: Kelp, celery, seafood, and sea salt supply sodium. Oranges, bananas, meat, dried fruit, melon, and vegetables supply potassium. Seafood, kelp, celery, pineapple, and meat supply chlorine.

Organically-bound Chromium is effective in regulating blood sugar levels.

Sources: Nutritional yeast, whole grains, liver, and mushrooms.

Iron deficiency is notorious for causing anemia. Although many of us consume potent tablets of iron, we remain anemic because the absorption of iron is difficult. Natural sources of iron are easier to assimilate. Vitamin C also promotes assimilation.

Sources: Liver, blackstrap molasses, nutritional yeast, egg yolk, dried apricots, sunflower seeds, and sesame seeds.

Selenium works closely with vitamin E as an anti-oxidant. It has also been found to help protect the body from mercury poisoning.

Sources: Nutritional yeast, kelp, whole grains, wheat germ, seafood, and eggs.

Fluorine should only be ingested in the form of calcium fluoride which is found in nature. Sodium fluoride which is added to our water supply and children's vitamins may be toxic. Fluorine is necessary for strengthening bones and teeth.

Sources: Seafood, sunflower seeds, almonds, and green vegetables.

Iodine is essential to the thyroid gland which controls energy levels, metabolism, physical and mental development.

Sources: Seafood, kelp, and egg yolk.

Manganese helps coordinate action between brain, nerves and muscles. It is important in the formation of human milk.

Sources: Whole grains, green leafy vegetables, kelp, wheat germ and bran.

Zinc promotes healing, aids in digestion, and is involved in carbohydrate metabolism. Deficiencies may appear as a loss of taste, poor appetite, retarded growth, and lethargy.

Sources: Sunflower seeds, pumpkin seeds, seafood, nutritional yeast, mushrooms, and organ meats.

Copper is necessary for the absorption of iron, protein metabolism, and for healing processes.

Sources: Organ meats, blackstrap molasses, nuts, and prunes.

Many other **trace minerals** exist whose functions in the human body are unknown or little understood. Using whole foods will guard against deficiencies.

Sources: Liver, nutritional yeast, kelp, seafood, seeds, sprouts, and basically all whole natural foods.

Overwhelmed?

If you feel overwhelmed by all this concentrated information you are not alone! This explanation of vitamins and minerals is merely to familiarize you with the range of vital nutrients you and your child will reap from foods when you commit yourselves to a new beginning.

Unwinding the Merry-Go-Round

A new beginning for your child and family revolves around a willingness to learn. We do not want our children to be less than the best they can be, yet many of us choose denatured food because it is convenient, available, and difficult to avoid at times. When reactions to chemicals and food become too overpowering to ignore, we rely on drugs to control the symptoms — but permit the cause to remain unchanged.

Some may argue that changing a child's diet to whole, natural food is too difficult and time-consuming. Parents may be discouraged by the lack of information available on *how* to establish truly nutritious food in children's diets. Many attempts to alter a child's diet fail because sugar is not eliminated, so the child continues to be vitamin B deficient. As long as a vitamin B deficiency exists, the child will crave sugar, blocking changes in eating habits.

Untangling your child's emotional and physical ties to junk food is not accomplished in one swift motion. The length of time necessary for your child's unwinding will depend upon:

¶ Previous eating habits.
¶ What deficiencies exist.
¶ Acceptance of new things.
¶ Peer group pressure.
¶ The example parents set.
¶ Siblings' attitude.
¶ Time spent watching TV.

¶ Availability of junk food.

¶ Your patience, enthusiasm, creativity, and confidence in learning with your child.

Each child will be unique in the transition to whole foods. For some children it will be a lengthy process; for others, the new step will be taken with ease. For all, it will be an ever-growing process.

The Way It Is

The food children eat varies from day to day in quantity and selection. Yet basic diets can be outlined in order for you to see where your child stands nutritionally. The following sample diets are on a scale of worst to passable. You may recognize your child's diet here. Or eating habits may fall somewhere in-between.

The Worst Diet

Example One

Example Two

BREAKFAST
Tang
Sugar cereal with milk
White bread toast

Two jelly donuts
Hot chocolate

LUNCH
Canned spaghetti
White bread and bologna
    sandwich
Kool-Aid
Twinkee

Instant cup of soup
Hot dog on a white bun
Jello
Hi-C

SNACKS
Candy bar
Potato chips

Snackin' Cake
Cherry popsicle

DINNER
TV dinner
White roll with butter
Chocolate milk
Ice cream

Macaroni and cheese from
    package
Applesauce containing sugar
French fries
Carbonated beverage

It's hard to believe that any child actually eats this way, but, unfortunately, far too many do. Parents who permit their children to eat like this convince themselves that this diet eliminates finickiness over food. Besides, it's cheap, convenient, and "enriched"! Parents who work, are overwrought, or simply don't realize the impact food has on health, fall prey to choosing sugary, fast foods.

The Mediocre Diet

Example One

BREAKFAST
French toast and syrup
Milk

LUNCH
Grilled cheese sandwich on rye bread
Potato chips
Milk

SNACKS
Oatmeal cookie (made with sugar)
Apple

DINNER
Spaghetti
Garlic bread
Salad with lettuce and tomato
Milk

Example Two

Oatmeal with milk and brown sugar
Sweetened orange juice

Taco
Burrito
Carbonated drink with artificial sweetner

Granola bar (made with sugar)
Ice cream

Fried chicken
Potato salad
Coleslaw
Apple Pie

A diet such as this is probably the most common. The parents understand the importance of the basic food groups; they try to balance the diet, more or less, but it still contains sugar, chemicals, and white flour. Often, parents are aware that sugar is not good, and keep a close watch on the sugar bowl, but continue to use it in moderation. Some junk food is kept in the house. In baking done at home, whole foods are often substituted for empty ingredients. Substituting artificial sweeteners for sugar is a frequent mistake in this household, since that is offering one harmful substance for another. If any type of granular sugar *must* be used, date sugar is the best transitional choice.

The Passable Diet

Example One	*Example Two*
BREAKFAST	
Egg	Buckwheat pancakes
Bran muffin	Sausage
Unsweetened orange juice	Milk
LUNCH	
Tuna sandwich with lettuce and tomato on whole wheat bread	Peanut butter and honey on whole wheat bread
Homemade soup	Orange
Apple juice	Milk
SNACKS	
Popcorn	Raisins
Banana	Granola
DINNER	
Steak	Fish
Fresh mashed potato	Fresh broccoli
Fresh zucchini	Fresh carrots
Fresh fruit salad	Milk
Milk	Gingerbread

This diet just about eliminates the ingestion of sugar, chemicals, and white flour. A mother who offers her child a diet like this is seriously interested in nutrition and the health of her family. However, this diet is not complete enough to insure excellent health. Take this diet, add more raw and concentrated food, and you'll have a superior diet for superior health.

The Forward Movement

Changing your child's eating habits is a slow, transition process. The following examples are guidelines for a new beginning with food for your child. The transition has been separated into four parts but this should, by no means, be viewed as the exact way and sequence for your child. For instance, some children love yogurt from the start, while others have to develop a taste for it.

Do not try to introduce your child to new foods by allowing some that contain chemicals or refined sugar, such as yogurt with sugar instead of honey. This will be confusing later when you try to remove them.

Let your child take the lead, and easy does it with the whole procedure on your part.

On the Way Up from Rock Bottom

If your child is seriously addicted to empty food, do not despair! With a finicky, sugar-addicted child, begin with a diet that works around favorite foods.

Goodies are very important to this child, so include some in the new diet: Simply *substitute nutrient-rich products for empty ones.* Some brands of luncheon meats, ice cream sandwiches, animal cookies, licorice, naturally carbonated drinks, cake mixes, chili, and whole wheat noodles are now available without sugar or chemicals. Every day something new pops up on the market that makes it easier for us to live in a fast food world — *naturally.* And there are endless possibilities of nutritious things you can make yourself to please the taste of a sweet-oriented child — muffins, candy apples, peanut brittle. With the right ingredients, these goodies build health, while your child gradually develops new tastes.

So, the first step toward your child's new beginning is a trip to the health food store to find out what is available. Experimenting in the kitchen is the next step . . . and you're on your way!

FIRST STEP SAMPLE DIET

Example One
BREAKFAST
One-eyed Texan — cut round
    hole in whole wheat bread
    and place egg in center
Carob milk, hot or cold
Whole orange

LUNCH
Bologna sandwich — bologna
    without chemicals,
    cheese, touch of avocado,
    lettuce
Homemade soup   Apple

Example Two

Egg
Sausage (made from turkey
    or beef without chemi-
    cals)
Honey granola with fruit and
    milk

Quick Chili*
Natural corn chips
Carbonated apple juice
Fruit salad

---

* Recipes in Chapter Thirteen.

SNACKS
Health Valley [brand name]
  beef jerky
Fruit kabob

DINNER
Spaghetti — DeBole [brand
  name] artichoke spaghetti noodles, meat sauce
  spiked with grated vegetables, and topped with
  lots of cheese
Coleslaw or salad with natural dressing*
Milk
Honey Custard*

Natural Nector Ice Cream
  Sandwich

Macaroni and Cheese De-
  luxe*
Carrots Glazed with Honey*
Raw Applesauce*
Natural grape gelatin (grape
  juice, gelatin, and water)
Milk

Inching Along
  The next step, after introducing some new tastes, is establishing some concentrated foods in the diet. Muffins, milkshakes, meatloaf, crackers, and cookies are good foods to spike
with nutritious substances. Go lightly at first. More raw foods
are also encouraged at this time in the form of raw fruit and
vegetables, salads, Smoothies** sandwiches, or Un-Sandwiches**.

SECOND STEP SAMPLE DIET

Example One

BREAKFAST
Honey Bran Muffins*
Fruit salad
Milk

LUNCH
Egg salad with Pizzazz** on
  sprouted wheat bread
Natural orange gelatin with
  grated carrot and pineapple
Milk

Example Two

Power Pancakes** with real
  maple syrup
Whole orange
Milk

Whole wheat tortilla grilled
  with avocado, cheese, tomato, sprouts*
Homemade soup
Smoothie**

* Recipes in Chapter Thirteen.
** Recipes in Chapter Two.

SNACKS
Trail mix
Carob popsicles (freeze Mar-
    velous Munchkin Mix**)

Celery stuffed with almond
    butter
Carob Chip Cookie*

DINNER
Chicken with a Crunch*
Confetti Salad*
Yams
String beans with sliced al-
    monds
Milk

Happy Hot Dogs*
Potato Pancakes*
Broccoli
Carrot Cake*
Milk

New Sensations

As your child and you continue to grow nutritionally,
increase the concentration of nutrients in food, and introduce
more new taste sensations. At this stage you should notice much
improvement in your child's health and in your own well-being!

THIRD STEP SAMPLE DIET

Example One

BREAKFAST
Egg
Nutty Muffin*
Pineapple chunks
Milk

Example Two

Marvelous Munchkin Mix**
Homemade Granola* with fruit

LUNCH
Chicken thigh or drumstick
Fresh-squeezed orange juice
Yogurt with sunflower seeds
    and banana
Bronners [brand name] corn
    chips
Carob Brownie*

Peanut butter (add yeast, rai-
    sins, honey, milk powder)
    on multi-grain bread
Carrot-Raisin Salad*
Milk
Gingersnaps*

---

* Recipe in Chapter Thirteen.
** Recipe in Chapter Two.

SNACKS
Frozen banana
Vegetables with dip

Finger Gelatin***
Dried fruit

DINNER
Special Burgers* with
    sprouts, cheese, tomato
    on whole wheat bun
Potato Salad*
Milk

Lots of Lasagna*
Salad with sprouts, avocado,
    spinach, etc.
Raw Applesauce*
Gingerbread*

Growing on Course

Moving in the right direction is fairly easy once you get started. Keep the foods you prepare attractive and exciting as much as possible. If your child enjoys working in the kitchen, let your child prepare a meal, or bake a special surprise.

FOURTH STEP SAMPLE DIET

Example One

Example Two

BREAKFAST
Egg
Cottage cheese
Honey Bran Muffin*
Fresh-squeezed orange juice

Seed Pancakes* with real maple syrup
Sausage (beef or turkey without chemicals)
Smoothie**

LUNCH
Cucumber boats — filled
    with Tuna Salad with Pizzazz** and topped with
    sprouts
Juicy Delight**
Seed Crackers*

Pita sandwich — avocado,
    meat, cheese, tomato,
    sprouts on whole wheat
    Pita bread
Carrot/orange juice
Seed Cookies II*

SNACKS:
Cheese
Seeds and nuts

Yogurt
Dried apricots

---

* Recipes in Chapter Thirteen.
** Recipes in Chapter Two.
*** Recipe in Chapter Twelve.

DINNER

Meat Loaf Supreme**	Shrimp-avocado-cheese om-
Salad (as many different veg-	elet
gies as you can think of)	Sautéed mushrooms
Asparagus	7-grain English muffin
Kefir milk	Fresh fruit
	Milk

These diets gradually increase the quantity of nutritious substances. Your child's diet will probably fluctuate from day to day. All the food listed in the transition sample diets are nutritious, but you should work toward the addition of raw and concentrated food.

Depending upon the age and nutritional needs of your child, the quantities of food you offer will vary. Keep portions of new food small and, where possible, introduce them with other foods until a taste has developed. For instance, put yogurt in Smoothies**, icing, salad dressing, or serve as ice cream (frozen yogurt) before offering it plain.

Your new beginning may go more smoothly if you talk to your child about the coming changes in diet. If your child is severely addicted to sugar or is very young, this communication will need to wait until acceptance or maturity makes it possible. Once you get started, you and your child will learn in your own way and your own time.

** Recipes in Chapter Thirteen.

CHAPTER TWELVE

Food For A New Beginning

L earning to make *real* food a way of life isn't an easy, overnight process. To help you begin, I have broken down the how, what, which, where, and why of introducing nutritious food. Discovering new food is fun, but it can be frustrating if you don't know which foods to choose.

How To Change Empty Food into Nutritious Food

Most empty foods your child is accustomed to can be changed into nutritious food. Many can be purchased, but some will need to be made at home. As more people become concerned about eating healthfully, more foods that are fun *and* nutritious will be available. There is quite a trend already toward convenience in nutritious foods.

Buying Nutritious Food: Foods you make yourself, spiked with nutritious substances, are the most beneficial to your child. But if you want to purchase some things for convenience or a change of pace, the following products can be used in moderation as alternatives to empty food.

COOKIES, CAKE, AND PIE TO BUY

Animal cookies, an old favorite, are available from El Molino Mills, made with honey. Midel and Health Valley [brand names] both make a delicious graham cracker. You will find many kinds of cakes, pies, and cookies in health food stores, but check labels carefully for sugar. A natural food bakery in your town will offer the freshest and most nutritious snacks, if they are made only with honey. Health food stores often carry locally made natural desserts.

Here are some nutritious snacks that are widely available:

¶ Lifestream cookies — Strawberry, almond, raspberry delights!

¶ El Molino Mills — Bran, oatmeal, and peanut butter *honey* cookies. (Some of their products contain sugar.)

¶ Pride of the Farm — Date, peanut, oatmeal, carob, sesame, and gingerbread *honey* cookies. (Some of their products contain sugar.)

¶ Barbara's — Brownies, butter-nut cookies, macaroons, carrot cake, Russian tea cookies, etc. (Check labels; a few contain sugar.)

¶ Sovex — Granola, molasses, coconut, and peanut butter cookies.

¶ Healthway — natural cookies in many different flavors (check labels)

¶ Health Valley — Snaps and cookies at their best — Ten great kinds.

¶ Health Valley — Naturally good cakes.

¶ Natural Nector — Pies and cheesecake that taste great!

CANDY TO BUY

Much of the candy stocked in health food stores contains raw sugar. Avoid this type of candy. Raw sugar is used in candy (sometimes along with honey) to make it hard. Honey tends to yield a softer, chewier product.

Fructose is being used in some products now, but not widely, because it is more expensive. Burry's [brand name] and Caroba [brand name] have made available a complete line of carob products without sweetening such as carob bunnies and Santas, carob suckers, carob covered dried fruit and nuts as well as carob chips and bars.

You may find a local natural bakery that makes natural candy.

The following products in your health food store do not contain sugar:

¶ Naura Hayden's Dynamite bar — available in various flavors.

¶ Panda Licorice — Available as black and red licorice.

¶ Soken Plum Candy — Hard candy made from wheat syrup and plums.

¶ Soken Seaweed Candy — Chewy candy sweetened with wheat syrup.

¶ Tania's — Four kinds of outrageously good goodies (Raisin-Nut Crunch, Sesame-Coconut Chews, Apricot-Cashew Crunch, Maple-Nut Chews).

¶ Lifestream — Excellent line of candy with very nutritious ingredients (Sunshine Bar, Mega Bite, Hikers, Carob-Mint Fudge, Cashew Halvah, and Sesame Dream).

¶ Natural Halvah — Three flavors of halvah at its finest (ground sesame seeds and honey with Carob, Cashew-Currant, or Plain flavoring).

¶ Chico San Taffy and Caramels — Chewy candy sweetened with rice syrup.

¶ Golden Temple (Wha Guru Chew) — Three varieties of chewy, nutty bars (Original, Cashew-Almond, and Sesame-Almond).

¶ Lind Bars — Nutritious bars that are very good but may not appeal to the beginner.

¶ Queen Bee Taffy — Natural honey taffy in many flavors. This candy is very sweet; choose those that contain nuts.

¶ Nik's Treats — Hard candy in many delicious flavors.

¶ Burry's carob bars — Carob in mint, nut, crunch, plain.

ICE CREAM TO BUY

To meet the demands of the "I scream, you scream, we all scream for ice cream" crowd, Natural Nector† [brand name] has come out with natural honey ice cream novelties. Your family can enjoy:

¶ Ice cream sandwiches.

¶ Carob-fudge bars.

¶ Carob-coated vanilla bars.

¶ Ice cream between two granola cookies dipped in carob.

---

† Some of their products contain chocolate and sugar, check labels.

¶ Frozen yogurt between two granola cookies.

Shiloh Farms [brand name] also makes natural ice cream novelties, frozen yogurt, and natural popsicles. Make ice cream cones with Natural Cones [brand name] and honey ice cream or frozen yogurt. Be certain that the frozen yogurt is not filled with sugar and chemicals and that the natural ice cream does not contain sugar.

CRISPY, CRUNCHY, AND CHEWY SNACKS TO BUY

Whole grain crackers, chips, puffs, and pretzels are available and can be eaten in moderation.

Health Valley, Soken, Bronners, Barbara's, Hain, Chico San, and Erewhon offer a wide variety of chips and crackers you may wish to use:

¶ Cheese crackers
¶ Potato chips
¶ Pretzel twists and sticks
¶ Cheese puffs
¶ Tortilla chips
¶ Seaweed crackers
¶ Multi-grain crackers

¶ Whole wheat crackers
¶ Corn chips
¶ Vegetable crackers
¶ Yogurt chips
¶ Vegetable crackers
¶ Rice crackers
¶ Vege-Soy crackers

Chips with more nutritional value:

¶ Moo Munchies — Made with only milk powder and seasoning. The onion-flavored ones make excellent croutons.

¶ Tempah Chips — Made from soy that has been "predigested" by fermentation.

¶ Prothins — Protein chips available in various flavors (sea salted, barbecue, celery, onion).

¶ Bran-A-Crisp — High-bran cracker with a bit of rye flour.

¶ DeBole Sesame Artichoke Sticks — Bread sticks with gluten flour, artichoke flour, and sesame seeds.

Most of the following items contain more nutritional value and should be chosen over pretzels or potato chips:

¶ Dried beef sticks — Made without nitrates or nitrites by Health Valley.

¶ Dried fruit — Unsulfured, unsweetened fruit. Barbara's has a good crunchy dried apple product.

¶ Trail mix — Many varieties of trail mix are on the market, but my favorite is Westbrae's Sweet Nut Thins.

¶ Raw seeds and nuts — Stress seeds (they have more

minerals), but any nut your child enjoys is fine, too.

¶ Twinlab Crunchy Yogurt — A new taste treat that is expensive, but handy for nibbling. Comes in three flavors (plain, raspberry, and pineapple).

CEREALS TO BUY

Cereals need to be chosen carefully. Many of them have too many carbohydrates and little else. Those with wheat germ, milk powder, seeds, and nuts provide some protein, vitamins, and minerals. Multi-grain cereals are more nutritious than those containing mostly oats or wheat. Puffed cereals available from El Molino Mills (corn, millet, wheat, rice) are alright for a change, but are not a complete breakfast. You may try Erewhon Brown Rice Crispies or New World Raisin Bran.

The most nutritious cereals are made by:

¶ Arrowhead Mills   ¶ Health Valley
¶ Better Way   ¶ New World
¶ El Molino   ¶ Sovex
¶ Erewhon   ¶ Westbrae

BEVERAGES TO BUY

By far the best choice of beverages are fruit and vegetable juices. Fresh-squeezed is best, but, on occasions, you may wish to use carbonated juices.

Health Valley, Ocerola, R.W. Knudsen and Sons, and Dr. Tima all make carbonated sodas and juices.

Pure juices are available in bottles and/or cans from Westbrae, Hauiki, Heinke, and Lakewood. Wagner makes a natural fruit punch concentrate.

Making Your Own Nutritious Food: Many foods children enjoy are unavailable through health food stores. Making your own peanut brittle or marshmallows or gingerbread or caramel apples gives you the opportunity to vary your child's diet while powerpacking the snacks. Here are some ideas on how you can create your family's favorite snacks. There are more ideas in the recipe section of this book, but don't hesitate to try your own ideas!

Granola Bars

Mix 1 egg per cup of homemade Granola*. (If using store-bought granola, use ¼ cup seeds and ¾ cup granola.) Spread out in baking pan. Bake in moderate oven until firm. Slice into bars.

Popsicles

Fruit juices make great popsicles. Try adding a little vegetable juice also. Smoothie** or Marvelous Munchkin Mix**, frozen in popsicle molds, are delicious and nutritious.

Gum

Don't start the gum habit, but if it already exists, offer your child honeycomb to chew. It's a mother's delight because your child can swallow it!

Caramel Apples

Simmer 1½ cups of honey and ¾ cup cream over low heat until it reaches the soft ball stage. Mix with 2 T. butter. Cool mixture a bit, and beat in ½ cup non-instant milk powder. Dip apples and sprinkle with ground nuts.

Frozen Bananas

Cut bananas in halves and insert wooden sticks. Dip in Carob Syrup**, roll in ground nuts, and freeze.

Carob Syrup

Beat 2T. butter with 2T. carob powder and 1T. milk powder. Simmer in a saucepan with ¼ cup honey. Then stir in ½ tsp. vanilla. Serve hot. If syrup is to be served cold, add 1 or 2 T. milk to thin.

* Recipe in Chapter Thirteen.
** Recipes in Chapter Two.

SNOW CONES

Blend whole fruit and juice such as apples and apple juice. Freeze in ice cube tray and blend again until snowy.

NATURAL SODA

Add sparkling mineral water to any fruit juice.

SUN BRITTLE

Cook ½ cup honey to the hard ball stage (½ hour). Put 1 cup raw sunflower seeds in a buttered pan and pour hot honey over the seeds. Cool and break into pieces.

HOT (CAROB) CHOCOLATE

Blend 2 cups milk, ¼ cup carob powder, 2 T. honey, and a pinch of cinnamon. Heat slowly.

FROZEN YOGURT

Use plain yogurt and your own fresh fruit. Blend and freeze into popsicle molds.

NATURAL "SOME-MORES"

Melt homemade Marshmallows* over the campfire or your stove. Put between two graham crackers (Midel or Health Valley), with a slice of a Burry's [brand name] carob bar or Caroba [brand name] carob chips.

PLAY-DOUGH MIX

Mix 2 cups peanut butter (or a mixture of other seed and nut butters) with 1 cup honey. Knead in 4 T. nutritional yeast, ¼ cup wheat germ, and ½ cup milk powder or protein powder. Supply raisins, coconut, etc. for decorations. After the fun of making shapes, or probably during, your toddler can nibble at the play-dough.

---

* Recipe in Chapter Thirteen.

DOUGHNUTS

Combine ½ cup whole wheat flour, 2 T. nutritional yeast, 2 T. soy flour, ¼ cup seed flour, ¼ tsp. cinnamon, and 1 T. baking powder. Beat ¼ cup honey, ½ cup milk, 1 egg, and ¼ cup safflower oil and mix with dry ingredients. Bake in a doughnut machine.

MOCK CRACKER JACKS

Mix 4 cups popped popcorn, 1 cup peanuts, ½ cup sunflower seeds, ½ cup sesame seeds, ½ cup chopped almonds, and ¼ cup coconut. Melt 2 T. butter and coat the popcorn-nut mixture. Roast until coconut is light brown, then stir in popcorn and just enough honey and pure maple syrup to coat the mixture.

FINGER GELATIN

Soften 4 T. of gelatin in ¾ cup of orange juice. Boil 1 cup water and stir in orange juice mixture. Add ¼ cup honey and 1 cup carrot juice. Cool in 9-inch buttered pan and cut in squares when firm. For layered gelatin add homemade Marshmallow Fluff* and then an additional layer of gelatin.

FINGERPAINT

Any natural pudding* works well!

DOTS

Remember the little colored dots you would peel off paper to eat as a child? Make your own with natural ingredients! Boil 1 cup water and blend with 8 oz. of pure pectin in blender. Add a small can of frozen orange juice and blend well. Drop in tiny dots onto waxed paper and allow to dry thoroughly for a few days. This fun snack is from *The Natural Foods Blender Book*, by Frieda Nusz.

* Recipes in Chapter Thirteen.

Which Direction to Work Toward

Most of us would be shocked if brown or green spaghetti were set before us instead of the white variety we're accustomed to. Children are no different. You must introduce new foods a step at a time, working gradually toward the most concentrated and nutritious ones. Some steps may be skipped if your child has no past conceptions of how a particular food looks and tastes; the younger your child, the more steps can be skipped in changing diet.

This list may help you chart your progress from denatured foods to the most nutritious. Don't be discouraged if your child flatly refuses to cooperate with some of the foods you offer. We all hit plateaus where we resist taking the next step. Work with foods your child enjoys, spiking them lightly to develop a taste for the foods.

Breads: If you eat white bread exclusively in your home, your child will probably reject a whole grain bread. Begin with a light brown bread that contains ½ unbleached white and ½ whole wheat flour. Try your hand at homemade bread; it's hard to resist fresh, hot bread right from the oven. Move gradually toward darker, heavier breads.

Hamburger and Hot Dog Buns — Soy buns are light in color and are good to start with. Branch out with whole wheat or sprouted whole wheat buns.

Sandwich bread — Try different types of breads for sandwiches such as whole grain pocket bread, bran bread, whole grain tortillas, and various types of multi-grain breads.

Rolls — Start with the lighter variety of rolls (soy) and steadily work toward whole grain. If you make your own, the transition can be very gradual.

Tortillas — Your family may enjoy whole wheat burritos; multi-grain tortillas are also good.

Muffins and Biscuits — It is best to make these yourself so you can control the ingredients. Elf Liberty [brand name] has a nice packaged muffin mix that is handy, but add a few tablespoons of nutritional yeast to boost the B vitamin content. Sprouted 7-grain muffins and Wayfarers [brand name] bread (sprouted wheat or rye) are both excellent.

Dairy Products: Switching to raw, certified cow's milk is easy since there is no change in taste. It does taste fresher, so your child may drink more.

Since so many children are allergic to cow's milk, you may want to try raw, certified goat's milk instead. Before you turn up your nose at the thought, know that very fresh goat's milk is delicious. The older it gets, however, the stronger and more "goaty" the flavor. My first taste of goat's milk was revolting; I tried everyting to kill the taste of it. I didn't realize I had drunk milk that was *not* fresh. Luckily, when I got up enough courage to try it again, I drank truly fresh milk. It is so delicious that my son and I now drink it by the quart. Goat's milk may not be your cup of tea; it is not essential. You and your child may like to try it, though, for the experience.

Since yogurt and kefir are pre-digested, they are much easier to handle than milk. If your child reacts to even yogurt, it could be a result of a lactose intolerance. This is a deficiency of the enzyme lactase which digests the sugar in milk. (Milk sugar is lactose.) Powder and tablets are available to supply the lactase enzyme your child may be lacking.

Milk — Try to obtain raw, certified cow's or goat's milk; if unavailable, acidophilus milk is your next best choice.

Yogurt — Don't use the sugar-laden, artificially colored and flavored variety. Choose honey-sweetened yogurt instead. The best of all is homemade yogurt or plain yogurt sweetened only with fresh fruit. Kefir is a liquid form of cultured milk that many children enjoy.

Ice Cream — The switch from sugar to honey is not noticeable if there is enough real flavor (from fruit, etc.). Ice cream or popsicles you make at home should be plain at first (without added nutrients) until new flavors are accepted. For instance, after your child has learned to enjoy popsicles made with plain juice, or milk and carob powder, then experiment a little with added nutrients.

Cheese — Use only natural cheeses that are not dyed or processed. Raw milk cheese is more expensive but worth every extra penny in taste and nutritional value.

Butter and Margarine — Buy only undyed butter and margarine. This will most likely be found in health food stores, but sometimes it is possible to find butter without dyes in a grocery store. Natural butter and cold pressed oil may be mixed to make "margarine."

Dry Milk Powder and Whey — The addition of these powders does not change the taste of drinks, puddings, cakes, etc., because they simply taste like milk.

Eggs — Add eggs wherever possible. An egg added to fresh orange juice and blended on high makes a delicious, foamy drink. Add an egg to milkshakes without a change in taste.

Seasonings: Most of us consume a heavy amount of salt, a habit which we pass on to our children. Switching to sea salt is the first step, but not the answer. Learn to use more herbs and spices for seasoning instead of salt. Vegetable salt is a good transition seasoning, but eventually you will find that salting food is really not necessary. In our home the salt shaker is filled with kelp.

Steak sauce, meat marinade, barbeque sauce, catsup, bouillon, mayonnaise, salad dressing, mustard, seasonings for meat loaf, meatballs, and Sloppy Joes made without sugar or chemicals are now available in health food stores.

Sweetenings: Toss the sugar bowl into the garbage can and replace it with the honey pot. Date sugar may be used to replace brown sugar. Raw honey, blackstrap molasses, and maple syrup are preferable sweeteners; use in moderation, decreasing the quantity of sweetening used in recipes gradually. Bee pollen may be used to sweeten cereals and candy.

Pasta: Begin with soy, artichoke, or sesame noodles and spaghetti. Darker pastas, like dark green spinach noodles, may not be accepted right away. Whole wheat alphabets shouldn't produce much of a problem. For allergy to wheat use corn or rice pasta.

Gelatin: If your child likes gelatin, begin with fruit juices and progress to vegetable juices or combinations of fruit and vegetable juice. Try Hain Gel Dessert [brand name].

Cereals: Getting your child off sugar cereals and onto natural cereals is not an easy task since the choice of natural cereals just isn't there. Let's face it — sugar cereals are convenient, and one of the few breakfasts that your child can fix alone.

It may be a good idea to ease up on breakfasts based on cereal, and introduce some new breakfast ideas. If you are rushed for time in the morning, or if your child must manage alone, there are many quick, nutritious foods. Muffins, milkshakes, yogurt with fruit, and Smoothies** are all quick and easy. So are hardboiled eggs, tuna salad, fruit, or whatever else tickles your child's fancy.

Make your own granola to insure highly nutritious ingredients*. To avoid rejection of granola, don't introduce it as a cereal. Use it to make granola bars, as a topping on ice cream, in cookies, or possibly as a snack by itself.

Hot cereals such as millet, buckwheat, and soy may not go over too well, so add dried fruit, cinnamon, and honey.

Cereals should be liberally spiked with nuts, milk powder, wheat germ, bran, and ground seeds to balance the high carbohydrate content.

Protein: As the price of meat soars, many families are eating less meat and more fish, poultry, and even a few vegetarian dishes now and then. Organ meats are the most nutritious, yet getting children to eat liver is difficult, if not impossible. Adding ground liver to mashed potato or to meatloaf (small amounts at first) mellows out the taste and helps to develop a taste for it. Strangely, many people who hate liver really enjoy liverworst. Give it a try with your child if you can obtain it without chemicals. To decrease saturated fat in a diet, you can switch from pork sausage to turkey sausage.

Nuts and Seeds: If raw seeds and nuts are rejected, roast them yourself. (Spread on cookie sheet, brush with butter, and put in low heat oven for an hour or two.) Begin adding raw nuts and seeds to the roasted ones, increasing proportions gradually.

Fruits and Vegetables: Fruits are usually well received by children; it's vegetables that cause the trouble. The starting point with vegetables is whatever your child will accept in whatever form. If rejection is strong for any food that has anything to do with vegetables, sneaking may be in order.

Goodies: At first you may need to rely on goodies from the health food store. As you become more confident in making your own goodies, work toward making them more nutritious.

---

* Recipe in Chapter Thirteen.
** Recipe in Chapter Two.

Where To Find Nutritious Food

If you have been wondering what you can buy at the supermarket after steering clear of food containing sugar and/or chemicals, the answer is — not much. Greater public awareness has resulted in slightly reduced use of chemicals in foods. But sugar is still omnipresent at the supermarket. Still, there are some *real* foods at the supermarket; it may take some searching to uncover them.

What you purchase at the supermarket will depend upon what is available at your local health food store or co-op. For instance, if it is hard or impossible to obtain certified, raw milk where you live, you will have to purchase milk from a dairy or from the supermarket.

Every health food store has its own character, since the people who own and work in them have different ideas about nutrition. Some stores tend to be sterile, with clerks dressed in white tunics, and deal mostly with vitamins. Others offer mostly bulk foods and produce, while still others balance between the two extremes. Visit all the health food stores in your area to find one that best suits your needs. Chain health food stores carry so many gimmicks and sugary, chemical-laden foods that they should not be allowed to associate themselves with health or nutrition.

Please remember that everything in a health food store, chain or not, may not be natural. Some health food stores are very strict about stocking only foods which build health; others are inexperienced and carry many products with sugar and/or chemicals. *Always read labels* unless you are familiar with what you are buying.

If your health food store does not carry something you want, speak to the person who does the ordering. Don't feel timid asking for a particular product; you are helping the store (and others) by getting it to carry a good product.

A local farmer can provide you with nutritious food that is fresh and inexpensive. If you can locate a farmer who is careful about what he feeds his animals and puts into his soil, you will be fortunate indeed.

Growing your own food is an excellent way to feed your family. Children who hate vegetables often change their minds when they help grow them in their own gardens, and then taste the superior flavor.

What Health Foods or Natural Foods Are

You will want to become familiar with many of the following new foods. It is not necessary to rush out and buy all these foods, but, eventually, you should get around to trying them all, and discovering which ones appeal to your family.

Arrowroot Powder: Nutritious substitute for cornstarch, processed without chemicals.

Agar-Agar: Vegetable from the sea that can be used as gelatin. Available in powder, flakes, and sticks.

Bee Pollen: Power-packed sweetener, loaded with B vitamins, minerals, and enzymes. Use in drinks, on cereals, in candy.

Bran: The outer coating of grains. Supplies beneficial roughage in the diet.

Brown Rice: Whole, unadulterated grain preferable to polished white rice. Long grain rice is light and fluffy when cooked; short grain is tender and moist.

Blackstrap Molasses: The mineral-rich part of cane or beet sugar which is spun off in the refining process. High in B vitamins and iron. Do not give directly from spoon to your child because it sticks to the teeth.

Brewers Yeast: Also known as nutritional yeast. A powerhouse of minerals and B vitamins. If you had to choose one nutritious addition, this would be it. Always begin with a tiny amount (½ tsp.) and work up slowly. If gas forms in the stomach, it is a sign of B vitamin deficiency. Don't discontinue the yeast, but reduce amount, and work up more slowly. Purchase only yeast which is balanced with calcium and magnesium (Donsbach Yeast 500 or Twinlab Super Yeast). Not to be confused with live bakers yeast.

Carob Powder: Powder ground from pods of the carob tree (St. John's Bread). Tastes very similar to chocolate without the bitterness and bad effects of chocolate. Low in fat, rich in minerals and natural sugar.

Desiccated Liver: Beef liver dried at low heat to retain valuable nutrients. Choose only that prepared from Argentine beef liver to guard against toxins. Use in tiny amounts because of strong flavor.

Dried Fruit: Natural dried fruit without chemicals and sweeteners is darker and drier than sulfured fruit. The taste is so delicious, the color is never missed. Try making your own!

Food coloring: Use Earth Grown, natural coloring or natural colors from fruits and vegetables.

Grains: Millet, one of the most nutritious, can be used as a cooked cereal or in casseroles. Wild rice and buckwheat are also very nutritious.

Granola: Crunchy cereal containing oats, wheat germ, nuts, and honey. Very nutritious if made at home, adding milk powder, seeds, soy flakes, etc.

Herbal Teas: Healthful blends of herbs, plants, and roots, legendary for curing and soothing various ailments. A wide variety awaits your discovery. Mix the more nutritious teas (comfrey, alfalfa) with the pleasant tasting ones (peppermint, spearmint). Try iced herbal tea for your child if he does not care for hot tea.

Honey: Raw, unfiltered honey is not as easily obtained as one might think since honey can be labeled as unheated if it has not been heated over 160°. Choose honey carefully to avoid those that are not really raw.

Honeycomb: Natural chewing gum that children can swallow!

Kelp: Sea vegetable that supplies many trace minerals. Use as seasoning on food in small amounts (strong tasting).

Kefir: Cultured milk similar to yogurt in liquid form. Cheese made from kefir tastes like cream cheese with fewer calories (kefir cheese).

Lecithin: Derivative of the soy bean that acts as an emulsifier in the bloodstream. Helps maintain a healthy nervous system and cleanses the liver and kidneys. Available in granules, liquid, and powder.

Legumes: Try as many different legumes as possible so that you can find the ones your family likes best. Lentils, azuki beans, mung beans, and soy beans are good choices.

Low Sodium Baking Powder: That which is free of sodium and aluminum compounds.

Milk Powder: Dried, *non-instant* powder that can be added to baked goods, cereals, puddings, and milkshakes to boost protein and mineral content.

Nuts: In their raw state, nuts taste differently than the roasted, salted, and usually rancid variety. Almonds, cashews, walnuts, and pecans are all good for snacking or as nut butters or flours.

Oils: Unrefined, cold-pressed oils (such as safflower and soy) supply essential fatty acids necessary for the structure of every body cell. Natural mayonnaise, salad dressing, nuts, avocado, and seeds provide oils in the diet. Any increase in oil must be accompanied with additional vitamin E. Some oils have extra vitamin E added; in wheat germ oil, it is naturally present.

Protein Powders: Most contain a mixture of soy, milk and/or egg protein. Six dollars or more per pound is a ridiculous price to pay for milk powder, dried eggs, and soy protein! Choose only a protein powder that contains glandular protein, yeast, lecithin, and other nutritive factors not in the usual diet. Make your own protein powder, mixing proteins you prefer. (Dr. Donsbach Gland-Pro or Naura Hayden's Dynamite protein powder may be used.)

Raw Fruits and Vegetables: Essential for enzymes, vitamins, minerals, roughage, and natural sugar. Try new fruits and vegetables with your child, instead of sticking to the same old apples and oranges. Make and combine juices from fresh fruits and veggies. Has your child ever tasted guava juice, or eaten a kiwi or an artichoke?

Real Maple Syrup: Most commercial brands contain 2 percent maple syrup, the remaining 98 percent is chemicals and sugar. Introduce real maple syrup into your home. Some taste differently than others — choose Canadian maple syrup over American, and Grade C over Grade A, because it contains more minerals.

Rice Polish: Outer coating of brown rice, contains a high quantity of B vitamins. Use in baking or add to cereals.

Rose Hips: Seeds at the base of rose blossoms, high in vitamin C and bioflavinoids. Use as herbal tea or as a vitamin supplement in powder, tablet, or liquid form.

Seeds: Seeds supply protein, minerals, vitamins, and unsaturated fatty acids. Ground seeds can be made into butter or used as flour in baking recipes. Sesame, sunflower, chia, and pumpkin are all nutritious additions to any food you prepare. Refrigerate all ground seeds. Ground seeds are referred to as *seed flour* in recipe section.

Sea Salt: Salt derived from sea water. Use sparingly, only in recipes where crucial. Salt should not be in a shaker, but tucked away in a box in your pantry.

Sprouts: Tremendously nutritious, sprouted grain and seeds supply raw vegetables all year round. Alfalfa sprouts are becoming very popular in place of lettuce on sandwiches. Health food and grocery stores carry sprouts, but growing your own in a three-tiered sprouter encourages children to taste what they have grown. Try alfalfa, mung, lentil, wheat, sunflower or any others in your sprouter or a mason jar with a cheesecloth covering.

Tofu: Soft cheese made from soy that is very bland in flavor. Use in casseroles, salads, or in place of regular cheese.

Unflavored Gelatin: Pure gelatin, easy and quick to use. Available in bulk or in packages. One tablespoon of gelatin equals one packet.

Variety Flours: Millet, rice, soy, wheat germ, nutritional yeast, milk powder, ground seeds, ground nuts. Flour need not be derived exclusively from wheat. Until you are at ease with using other flours, start out slowly, using ¾ wheat flour and ¼ variety flours. Whole wheat flour comes two ways. Pastry flour is used for cookies, cakes, pie crusts; regular whole wheat flour is used for baking bread.

Wheat Germ: The germ of wheat that contains a very high percentage of vitamins and minerals. Wheat germ must be fresh because it becomes rancid ten days after being milled. Use special care to guard against rancidity. Obtain wheat germ fresh from a mill and freeze a portion of it. Fearn [brand name] has a vacuum sealed wheat germ that is acceptable if fresh is unavailable.

Whey: The liquid left over when cheese is made. This nutritious milk product is usually thrown out, yet it supplies a high quantity of vitamins and minerals. Beneficial to the growth of friendly bacteria in the intestines.

Whole Grain Pasta: Spaghetti, lasagna, alphabets, noodles, macaroni, etc. are available in health food stores in whole grain form. DeBole [brand name] pastas use artichoke flour which is more expensive, but worth the cost, since it cuts back on the amount of starch in the pasta. Other pastas are made with buckwheat, corn, whole wheat, sesame, soy, and vegetable powders.

Yogurt: Cultured milk with a consistency like pudding. This predigested milk must be purchased in a health food store or made at home to avoid the sugar, coloring, and flavoring in the supermarket variety. Some supermarkets may carry natural yogurt in their health food department.

Why — The Inevitable Question of All Children

Your child is bound to approach you with questions about why natural foods are served in your home. Express your desire for the family to grow together nutritionally and help each other achieve the best of health.

Why? *Because the human body has requirements for nutrients that must be met before one can achieve mental, physical, and emotional well-being.*

The answer is there. You need only to reach for it . . . .

CHAPTER THIRTEEN

Recipes:
Main Dishes

The proteins in main dishes — like beef, turkey, chicken, natural cheeses, eggs — are fine for your child's new diet, and will not require any big changes or substitutions. Those containing nitrates or nitrites, such as salami, hot dogs, bologna, and bacon, can be purchased without contaminants in health food stores.

Starches will change somewhat. Alter favorite recipes by adding wheat germ instead of bread crumbs, brown rice instead of white, whole grain noodles instead of pasty ones, and concentrated ingredients instead of empty ones.

LOTS OF LASAGNA!

---

12 oz. whole wheat lasagna
1 lb. ground turkey or beef
½ cup shredded vegetables
¼ cup mushrooms
20 oz. spaghetti sauce (buy in a health food store or make your own)
2 cups cottage cheese
½ lb. jack or cheddar cheese
½ lb. Mozzarella cheese

Sauté ground meat and mushrooms, then add grated vegetables and spaghetti sauce. Cook noodles in boiling water until tender. Blend cottage cheese with a bit of milk until smooth.

Grate cheeses. In a large baking dish or pan alternate layers of
the above ingredients beginning with the cooked noodles, then
the sauce, then the cottage cheese, and then a sprinkling of each
grated cheese. Bake at 350° for about 40 minutes. Serves four
to six people.

Pizza A La Natural

2 cups Fearn [brand name] Soy-O whole wheat pancake mix
½ cup wheat germ
½ cup sunflower seed flour
2 T. nutritional yeast
¼ cup milk powder
⅓ cup safflower oil
1 egg
¾ cup milk
2 cups spaghetti sauce (buy in health food store or make your
own)
½ cup grated vegetables
¼ cup mushrooms
½ lb. ground beef or slices of natural sausage
1 tsp. oregano
¼ tsp. basil
garlic powder to taste
½ lb. grated cheese

Preheat oven to 375°. Mix first five ingredients. Combine
oil, egg, and milk. Then add to flour mixture until dough forms
a smooth ball, adding more flour if necessary. Roll out dough
and place on an oiled pizza pan. Bake dough for 15 minutes and
allow to cool.

Combine sauce, grated vegetables, garlic powder, basil, and
oregano. Spread mixture onto cooled pizza crust. Add cooked
ground beef or sausage and grated cheese. Bake at 375° for
about 30 minutes.

Special Burgers

½ cup Fearn [brand name] Sesame Burger Mix
½ lb. ground beef or turkey
1 egg — whole wheat buns
tomato sauce to moisten — sprouts
cheese slices — avocado

Form burger ingredients into patties and cook as you would regular hamburgers, except it will be necessary to coat the pan with a bit of oil. Serve on buns with slices of avocado and garnish with sprouts.

HOT TUNA

7 oz. can water-packed tuna
2 eggs
¼ cup sautéed mushrooms
⅓ cup grated cheese
½ cup cooked soy noodles
¼ cup ground seeds
¼ cup fresh or frozen peas
pinch of garlic
splash of milk

Mix all ingredients and top with cheese or wheat germ. Bake at 350° for about 40 minutes.

HAPPY HOT DOGS

4 slices whole grain bread
6 natural hot dogs (Health Valley [brand name] or other)
2 avocados
tomato slices
cheese slices
alfalfa sprouts
mayonnaise or natural dressing

Spread slices of bread with mayonnaise. Add avocado, hot dogs sliced lengthwise, tomato, and top with cheese. Bake in hot oven until cheese is bubbly. Garnish with sprouts and serve immediately.

MACARONI AND CHEESE DELUXE

2 cups soy macaroni
½ cup blended cottage cheese
¼ cup yogurt
2 T. ground wheat germ
½ cup jack or cheddar cheese
1 egg
½ cup milk

Cook macaroni in boiling water until tender. Blend egg, milk, soy powder and wheat germ. Mix together all ingredients and bake at 375° for 30 minutes.

Chicken with a Crunch

Melted butter or margarine   ¼ cup wheat germ
¼ cup whole wheat flour   ¼ cup whole sesame seeds

Dip chicken pieces in melted butter. Combine dry ingredients and add Spike [brand name] seasoning if desired. Roll chicken in coating and bake as usual.

Quick Chili

2 cans Health Valley [brand name] mild chili
½ cup grated cheese
4 natural hot dogs, cut up (optional)
1 T. nutritional yeast

Heat for a quick meal and serve with salad and Corn Bread*.

Grilled Tortillas

whole wheat tortillas   tomato
avocado   sprouts
cheese

Butter one side of a tortilla. Fill ½ other side with avocado, cheese, tomato, and sprouts. Fold it in half. Grill tortilla until brown on both sides.

Raw Fruits and Vegetables

Fruits and vegetables should be offered raw as much as possible in salads, soup, gelatin, or as snacks. Cut fruits and vegetables into interesting shapes and use a dip your child enjoys. Before-dinner munchies can be a plateful of raw vegetables. Be ready with a plate of raw fruits and vegetables for an anytime snack.

THE CREATIVE SALAD

Salad is not just iceberg lettuce and tomato! A real salad is one that changes from day to day. Add anything fresh. Create your own masterpieces with the addition of crumbled jack or cheddar cheese, seeds, toasted soy beans, Moo Munchies [brand name] for croutons (a chip made with milk powder instead of flour), and whatever else strikes your imagination. Don't hesitate to let your child have a turn at creating a salad.

Salad Makings:

asparagus	cucumber	parsley	spinach
avocado	eggplant	peppers	sprouts
broccoli	garlic	radishes	tomatoes
carrots	grated beets	raw peas	turnips
cauliflower	green cabbage	red cabbage	watercress
celery	mushrooms	romaine	zucchini
chard	onion		

RECIPES

Raw Applesauce

4 apples   1 tsp. honey (optional)
2 T. lemon juice   ½ tsp. cinnamon

Core and peel apples. Put all ingredients into the blender and blend until smooth.

Confetti Salad

Shred and combine any of the following in any combination.

Shred   *Add*

apple   carrots   coconut   almonds
beet   celery   pineapple   sesame seeds
cabbage   zucchini   raisins   walnuts

Gelatin Salad

Offer gelatin plain, with fruits, vegetables, nuts, or seeds. One pint of juice requires 1 T. of gelatin to set it.

½ cup boiling water
1½ cups juice (any except raw pineapple)
1 T. gelatin
1 cup of any shredded fruit or vegetable
¼ cup seeds or nuts

Melt gelatin in juice. Add boiling water and stir. Mix in any additions desired. Chill. Serve with a scoop of yogurt or whipped cream.

Carrot-Raisin Salad

1 cup shredded carrot   ½ cup crushed pineapple
¼ cup shredded apple   ¼ cup raisins
¼ cup shredded coconut   1 T. lemon juice

Mix and enjoy!

Super Salad

lettuce
sprouts (start with a small amount)
tomato, chunked
avocado, cubed
cheese, shredded
strips of natural bologna (Health Valley [brand name] or other)
Thousand Island dressing (mix natural mayonnaise, Hain
[brand name] natural ketchup, hard boiled egg)

This salad seems to agree with the taste buds of many
children. Try it and see how it works for your family. Use a generous amount of dressing and mix it thoroughly with the salad.

Raw Vegetable Soup

Chop and blend together at high speed in blender tomato,
beets, onion, carrot, greens, potato, or any other vegetables. Add
natural vegetable bouillon for seasoning. Warm to serving
temperature and garnish with shredded cheese.

Avocado Soup

Blend 2 cups milk with ¼ cup milk powder. Blend avocado
(large) with a bit of the milk mixture. Slowly add remaining
milk, add shredded cheese and warm to serving temperature.

Cooked Fruits and Vegetables

Dishes made with cooked fruits and vegetables can be boosted nutritionally with seeds, nuts, cheese, milk powder, yogurt, eggs, nutritional yeast, and wheat germ.

APPLE DELIGHT

Core apples leaving the bottom intact. Fill centers with ground nuts or seeds, honey, and cinnamon. Bake at 350° for 30 minutes.

VEGETABLE SOUP

The fun of making soup lies in your own creativity. First, get out your largest pot. Use any available fresh vegetables and chop into small or medium pieces (whatever you prefer). To make the stock, blend fresh tomatoes and add vegetable bouillon (there are many varieties at the health food store). Throw everything into the pot, adding cubes of meat, if you wish. Make soup early on Saturday mornings, so it's handy for quick food during the weekend. Freeze portions of soup for handy lunches and dinners.

POTATO PANCAKES

3 cups cooked mashed potatoes
2 eggs
½ cup jack cheese   ¼ cup wheat germ
¼ cup seed flour   1 T. nutritional yeast
½ cup milk powder   ½ tsp. garlic powder
   Mix all ingredients. Fry or bake at 350° for about 15
minutes. Add a bit of milk if too thick. Diced fish or meat may
be added.

VEGETABLES DELUXE

   Steam large pieces of any fresh vegetable, such as corn on
the cob (cut in thirds), broccoli, carrots, zucchini, cauliflower,
sweet potato. Place steamed vegetables in a baking dish, top
with lots of cheddar and jack cheese, and broil until cheese is
bubbly. Serve at once.

GLAZE FOR CARROTS OR ACORN SQUASH

¼ cup margarine or butter   flavor with cinnamon or mint
¼ cup honey   sesame seeds
   Bake carrots or squash as usual in glaze. Sprinkle with
sesame seeds before serving.

POTATO SALAD WITH TOFU AND CHEESE

2 cups diced cooked potatoes (with skins left on)
1 cup diced tofu
1 cup diced cheddar or jack cheese
4 to 6 chopped hard boiled eggs
3 or 4 slices cooked (nitrate-free) bacon, crumbled (optional)
dressing made with ½ yogurt and ½ mayonnaise
4 T. Westbrae natural pickle relish (optional)
bit of natural mustard
   Mix all ingredients using amount of dressing needed for
desired consistency. Hain Old Fashioned [brand name] dry
dressing mix may be added to the yogurt-mayo mixture for
more flavor. The tofu, eggs, and cheese make this a great meal
in itself. And honestly, no one will guess that the tofu is present
because it looks and tastes like the potato in this salad.

Pineapple Yams

1½ cups cooked, mashed yams
½ cup crushed pineapple
1 egg
¼ cup shredded unsweetened coconut
¼ cup sesame seeds

Mix all ingredients except seeds. Use seeds as topping.

Cheesy Zucchini

2 lb. thinly sliced zucchini
¼ lb. mushrooms
½ cup cottage cheese
1 egg
½ cup jack cheese

Steam zucchini and sauté mushrooms. Blend cottage cheese with egg until smooth. Layer a baking dish with the zucchini, mushrooms, and cottage cheese. Top with jack cheese. Bake at 350° for about 45 minutes.

Zipping Up Starch Foods

Cereals and grains should supply a hearty amount of vitamins and minerals. Introduce new grains such as millet and wild rice in casseroles; it's less shocking than seeing a deeply colored side dish instead of the usual white rice or potato. Cereals are best created at home to insure variety and freshness.

CREATIVE GRANOLA

The "natural cereal" you find in the grocery store is a concoction of rolled oats and brown sugar, with a bit of raisins, wheat germ, and nuts thrown in. It's one step better than sugar-coated, candy cereals, but by no means offers a nutritionally adequate breakfast. Granola purchased in a health food store is of higher quality if honey is used instead of sugar, but it cannot compare to what you can make yourself. You'll find it's fun to make, and easy enough for your child to do. Granola is simply a matter of throwing lots of different ingredients together and coming out with a new cereal each time.

Granola Suggestions:

Cereals
rolled oats
wheat flakes
wheat germ
rye flakes
bran
soy granules
rice polish

Seeds and Nuts
sunflower seeds
chia seeds
sesame seeds
pumpkin seeds
walnuts
pecans
cashews
almonds

Powders and Spices
carob powder
milk powder
nutritional yeast
cinnamon
ginger
allspice
nutmeg

Dried Fruits
coconut shreds
chopped dates
dried pineapple
dried apricots
raisins
dried apples
chopped dried papaya

Mix in large bowl:

6 cups cereal in any combination, stressing flakes
2 cups milk powder
½ cup carob powder (optional)
1 or 2 T. nutritional yeast
1½ cups dried fruit
2½ cups seeds and/or nuts.

Set aside.

Combine:

½ cup honey
½ cup melted butter (or oil)
vanilla, cinnamon, or desired flavoring

Mix into dry ingredients with your hands until crumbly. Real maple syrup or blackstrap molasses may be used instead of honey as part, or all, of the sweetening. Bake for about 2½ hours (more or less according to the amount of crunchiness your family enjoys) at 225°.

SUPER CEREAL

Grind in a grinder or blender ¾ cup of any seeds or nuts (such as sesame, almond, chia, filberts, sunflower, pumpkin, cashews). Add ¼ cup raw wheat germ, ½ cup chopped dried fruit (such as apricot, date, pineapple) and ½ cup raisins. Serve with milk.

MILLET

Add 1 cup of millet to 1 quart of boiling water. Cook for ½ hour or until all water is absorbed. Millet can be served in this way with raisins for breakfast. Cook in broth and serve with mushrooms, onion, and cheese as a side dish for dinner.

BUCKWHEAT GROATS

Sauté 1 cup buckwheat groats in 1 T. safflower oil. Add 4 cups of water or broth and steam until water is absorbed, about 25 minutes.

WILD RICE

Cook ½ cup wild rice with 2 cups of water or broth. Simmer until water is absorbed, about 45 minutes.

Dips, Dressings, and Spreads

Dips and dressing can make or break the amount of raw food your child eats. If the dip isn't appealing the raw vegetables may go uneaten, and if the dressing isn't just right, then the salad is left untouched. Try different recipes to find the ones your child likes most and encourage your child to experiment with you.

Spreads are more nutritious if you make your own, but you may want to purchase the base for spreads like nut, seed, or peanut butter. The taste of nutritional yeast is absorbed by peanut butter, making it a good base for many spreads you prepare.

BASIC MAYONNAISE

---

2 egg yolks (room temperature)
1 tsp. sea salt
1 tsp. honey
¼ tsp. dry mustard
4 T. lemon juice
1½ cups safflower oil (room temperature)

Blend everything except oil. Add oil very slowly to egg mixture. Will keep one week in your refrigerator.

BASIC BUTTER SPREAD

½ lb. butter
¾ cup safflower oil with vitamin E
1 tsp. liquid lecithin
    Mix thoroughly and refrigerate.

NATURAL CHEESE SPREAD

8 oz. kefir cheese (or cream cheese)
¼ cup butter
½ lb. grated jack or cheddar cheese
    Combine kefir (or cream cheese) and softened butter, then
add grated cheese. Store in refrigerator.

CHEESE SPREAD SUPREME

1 cup cottage cheese
4 oz. cheddar cheese
4 oz. cream cheese

¼ cup ground sesame seeds
½ ripe avocado, mashed
3 T. chives

    Blend cottage cheese until smooth. Mix in all ingredients.

GARBANZO SPREAD

¾ cup cooked, mashed garbanzo beans
¼ cup ground sesame seeds or sesame butter
¼ cup grated cheddar cheese
½ tsp. garlic powder
lemon juice
    Mix all ingredients and thin to desired consistency with
lemon juice.

SUPER SPREAD

¾ cup peanut butter   1 cup honey
½ cup milk powder   ¼ cup ground sunflower seeds
2 T. nutritional yeast   ¼ cup ground sesame seeds
½ cup ground wheat germ
    Mix ingredients thoroughly and refrigerate. Part of the
peanut butter may be substituted with almond or cashew butter.

MOCK PEANUT BUTTER

    Add 1 T. nutritional yeast and ¼ cup sunflower or sesame
butter to each ¾ cup peanut butter, increasing gradually. Add
carob, raisins, nuts, seeds, wheat germ, and coconut for variation.

THOUSAND ISLAND DRESSING

1 cup homemade mayonnaise   shredded cheese
4 T. honey ketchup   natural pickle relish (Westbrae)
2 cooked, chopped eggs
    Mix all ingredients. The pickle relish gives this dressing a
stronger flavor. My family prefers not to use it, but many enjoy
its flavor.

TAHINI DRESSING

½ cup tahini (sesame butter)
¼ cup lemon juice
½ clove minced garlic
    Mix and thin with water if desired.

AVOCADO DRESSING

1 ripe, mashed avocado   2 T. lemon juice
1 tomato, finely chopped   4 T. safflower oil
2 T. cream cheese   pinch of garlic powder
    Mix. Add a bit of grated cheese on top of dressing.

CREAMY HERB DRESSING

½ cup yogurt
½ cup homemade mayonnaise
    pinch of each of the following — parsley, onion flakes, basil,
    rosemary, oregano, thyme.

Grind herbs in blender to form a dry powder. Mix herbs, yogurt, and mayonnaise.

Avocado Dip

Combine:

2 mashed avocados
1 chopped tomato
2 T. lemon juice

pinch of garlic powder
¼ cup shredded cheese

Yogurt Dip

Combine:
1 cup yogurt
3 T. chives
½ cup ground seeds
pinch of garlic

Bean Dip

Combine:
1 cup cooked mashed garbanzo beans
4 T. ground sesame seeds
3 T. lemon juice

Cottage Cheese Dip

Combine:
smoothly blended cottage cheese
¼ cup grated carrot
a few raisins

Sour Cream Onion Dip

Combine:
1 cup yogurt
½ cup sour cream
Hain Onion [brand name] dry soup mix to taste

Nut Butter Dip

Use peanut, cashew, almond, sunflower, or sesame butter as a dip.

Cookies, Crackers, Candy, and Custard

Munchy-crunchy, nutty-chewy, and drippy-dippy snacks are essential to the fun of eating for children. These foods need to offer superior nutrients instead of being worthless fillers that spoil appetites. Bake with your child and discover new recipes that appeal to your family's taste buds. Cookies are excellent for children to create — more flour can be added if the batter is too moist, and more liquid if the batter is too dry. I had had three failures trying to create Seed Cookies II when my son decided to help me. I was in no mood to have any help, but he climbed up on a chair and started mixing things by himself. As I mulled over my failures, I half-heartedly watched my son mash a banana, add some honey, mix in an egg, and toss in some carob powder. When he asked me for some flour, it suddenly dawned on me that Seed Cookies II had been created before my eyes. Don't restrict yourself or your child with a recipe — *change it, vary it, experiment with it!*

PEANUT BUTTER COOKIES

¾ cup peanut butter
⅔ cup honey or real maple syrup
½ cup butter
1 egg, beaten
½ cup whole wheat pastry flour
2 T. nutritional yeast

1 cup seed flour
¼ cup milk powder
½ cup wheat germ
1 tsp. vanilla

Cream peanut butter and honey or maple syrup. Beat in butter and add egg. Mix dry ingredients and add to the peanut butter mixture. Add vanilla. Form into balls and flatten with the bottom of a glass. Place on oiled cookie sheet. Then bake for 20 minutes in a preheated oven at 325°.

NUT COOKIES

1 cup ground almonds
1 cup ground pecans
2 eggs
⅓ cup honey
1 tsp cinnamon

Mix eggs and honey. Stir in nut flours, then cinnamon. Drop onto oiled baking sheet and bake at 325° for about 20 minutes.

GINGERSNAPS

½ cup molasses
¼ cup honey
¼ cup safflower oil
1 egg
2 T. nutritional yeast
½ cup whole wheat pastry flour

½ cup seed flour
½ cup wheat germ
½ cup milk powder
1 tsp. cinnamon
1 tsp. ginger
1 tsp. cloves

Beat molasses, honey, and oil. Add egg. Mix dry ingredients and add to molasses mixture. Drop onto oiled baking sheet and bake for about 15 minutes at 350°.

TOP OF THE STOVE COOKIES

1¼ cup whole wheat flour
¼ cup wheat germ
1 cup milk powder
2 T. nutritional yeast
½ tsp. baking powder
¼ tsp. baking soda

½ tsp. nutmeg
½ cup butter
1 egg
½ cup honey
¼ cup milk
½ cup raisins

Mix dry ingredients, then cut butter into dry mixture. Beat egg, honey, and milk, then combine with dry ingredients and butter. Stir in raisins. Roll out dough on a floured board and cut dough ¼ inch thick with a two-inch cookie cutter. Cook on a lightly oiled griddle until lightly browned.

Carob-Almond Granola Squares

½ cup honey
¼ cup molasses
½ cup almond or peanut butter
2 eggs
1 T. nutritional yeast

¼ cup butter
3 cups homemade granola
¼ cup carob powder
½ cup chopped almonds

Mix honey, molasses, and butters. Add eggs and mix in remaining ingredients. Spread in 9-inch pan and bake at 350° for about 20 minutes. Cool and cut into squares.

Seed Cookies I

1¼ cups seed flour
1 cup shredded coconut

½ cup honey
1 egg

Combine and drop onto an oiled baking sheet. Bake at 300° for ½ hour.

Seed Cookies II

½ cup honey
2 mashed bananas
1 egg

1 cup seed flour
¼ cup carob powder

Mix honey, mashed banana, and egg. Mix dry ingredients and add to banana mixture. Drop onto an oiled baking sheet and bake at 300° for ½ hour.

Carob Chip Cookies

½ cup butter
⅓ cup honey or real maple syrup
2 eggs
½ cup carob chips (Caroba unsweetened carob chips)
½ tsp. baking powder

¾ cup milk powder
¼ cup seed or nut flour
½ cup wheat germ

Cream butter and honey. Add beaten eggs. Mix dry ingredients and add to honey mixture. Drop by teaspoon onto a buttered baking sheet. Bake at 350° for about 20 minutes.

OATMEAL-RAISIN COOKIES

1 cup honey	½ cup milk powder
½ cup safflower oil	1 tsp. nutritional yeast
1 egg	¼ tsp. cloves
2 cups rolled oats	½ tsp. nutmeg
¼ cup wheat germ	1 tsp. cinnamon
¼ cup seed flour	½ cup raisins
½ cup whole wheat pastry flour	

Mix liquid and dry ingredients separately and then combine. Stir in raisins. Drop by teaspoons onto an oiled baking sheet. Bake at 350° for 15 minutes.

SEED CRACKERS

½ cup ground sunflower seeds	½ cup shredded coconut
½ cup ground sesame seeds	¼ cup water
1 T. nutritional yeast	

Mix ingredients and knead into a ball. Flatten onto an oiled baking sheet, then roll very thin with waxed paper on top. Score dough and bake for about 45 minutes at 325°. Serve with peanut butter and a bit of banana on top.

SUPER CRACKERS

½ cup water
¼ cup safflower oil
1 cup whole wheat pastry flour
½ cup seed flour
1 T. nutritional yeast
¼ cup soy flour or protein powder
1 tsp. sea salt
⅓ cup shredded cheddar cheese
½ cup sesame seeds

Blend water and oil. Combine dry ingredients and mix with oil mixture. Add cheddar cheese. Knead dough, adding more water if too dry, and more flour if too sticky. Flatten on an oiled baking sheet, sprinkle with sesame seeds, and cover with waxed paper to roll dough out evenly. Score dough, and bake at 325° for about 20-25 minutes. Turn off oven and allow crackers to continue drying until oven is cool.

FRUIT AND VEGETABLE LEATHER

Any fruit or vegetable may be pureed in the blender and dried, at the lowest possible temperature, in your oven overnight. A dehydrator is not necessary — but you may find this so much fun you will want to purchase one.

¾ cup pureed apple
½ cup pureed carrot
1 T. lemon juice
2 T. unsweetened coconut flakes (optional)
⅛ tsp. cinnamon

Spread mixture, as thinly as possible, onto a cookie sheet lined with plastic wrap or parchment paper. Keep mixture away from the edges. Place another sheet on top of the mixture and press with a spatula for a more even distribution, then remove. Dry about 8 hours on lowest possible heat in oven or in a dehydrator. Roll up and store, or eat on the spot!

MARSHMALLOWS

I had given up hope of ever finding a recipe for natural marshmallows until I found this one in *The Natural Foods Blender Cookbook*, by Frieda Nusz (Pivot 1966.)

Boil ¾ cup water in a saucepan. Meanwhile, mix 2 T. cornstarch (yes, I tried it with arrowroot and it didn't work) with ¼ cup water, then stir into the boiling water. Add the following to the hot mixture:

½ cup honey
1 T. vanilla
¼ tsp. almond flavoring

Allow to cool in the freezer until partially frozen.

Now blend 1 cup warm-to-hot water with 3 T. gelatin until fluffy. Add partially frozen mixture by spoonfuls and blend again. If mixture is too thick, add a bit of cold water. Add 1 tsp. baking powder for a fluffier mixture (optional). Pour mixture into a glass dish and allow to cool in the refrigerator.

When stiff and cool cut into shapes with small cookie cutters and coat with arrowroot powder. Spread on a cookie sheet to dry. It is important to let these dry for a few days to achieve a taste and texture much like commercial marshmallows. Store at room temperature in a paper bag (not plastic).

Marshmallow Fluff

Blend 2 egg whites. Add marshmallows until blender is ½ full. Blend and add ½ cup safflower oil. Blend again.

Use for ice cream topping, layered gelatin, etc.

SUNNY APRICOTS

1 cup dried apricots
½ cup ground sunflower seeds
wheat germ or coconut

Grind apricots and mix with seed flour. Form into sticks and roll in wheat germ or coconut.

HANDY CANDY

1 cup peanut butter
1 cup honey
½ cup carob powder
1 cup ground wheat germ
1 cup seed flour
½ cup milk powder
2 T. nutritional yeast

Mix honey and peanut butter. Knead with remaining ingredients and form into sticks. Wrap in waxed paper and store in refrigerator.

SES-SUN-ME CANDY

½ cup ground sunflower seeds
½ cup ground sesame seeds
¼ cup fine coconut shreds
¼ cup sesame seeds
1 T. safflower oil
1 tsp. vanilla
honey as needed

Mix all ingredients except honey. Knead mixture with enough honey so that candy will stick together. Form into sticks and balls. Wrap in wax paper and refrigerate.

SUPER PEANUT BRITTLE

¼ cup chopped almonds   ¼ cup chopped peanuts
¼ cup whole sunflower seeds   1 cup honey
¼ cup whole sesame seeds

Bring honey to a boil using low heat and continue cooking until it reaches the hard ball stage. (Drop a bit of honey into cold water to test if it forms a hard, stiff ball.) Oil baking sheet, sprinkle on seeds and nuts, and pour hot honey onto baking sheet. Cool and break into pieces.

HONEY CUSTARD

2½ cups milk   1 T. gelatin
4 eggs   1 tsp. vanilla
⅓ cup honey   nutmeg

Dissolve gelatin in a small amount of milk over low heat, then add remaining ingredients. Stir over medium-low heat until thickened. Pour into cups and dust with nutmeg. This custard is very easy to make since it is cooked on top of the stove and popped into the refrigerator. Vary it by adding ½ cup ground seeds, nuts, fruit, coconut shreds, mashed carrots, or cooked pumpkin.

LEMON PUDDING

1½ cups water
½ cup honey (or more, to taste)
3 T. arrowroot powder
¼ cup water
2 eggs
½ cup lemon juice

Bring 1½ cups water and the honey to a boil in a saucepan. Meanwhile, add arrowroot powder to ¼ cup water and mix well. Pour arrowroot mixture into the boiling mixture. Boil on low for about 5 minutes. Stir in eggs and cook for a few minutes on low heat. Stir in lemon juice and refrigerate.

Any fruit juice may be used in place of the lemon juice and chopped fruit may be added. Or try Hain Pudding Mix.

CAROB BANANA-NUT PUDDING

2 cups warm water
3 T. arrowroot powder
½ cup milk powder
1 banana
¼ cup carob powder
¼ cup honey
2 beaten eggs
chopped almonds

Blend warm water, arrowroot, and milk powder. Add honey, bananas, and carob powder. Heat in a saucepan, stirring constantly over medium-low heat until thick. Add beaten eggs and cook over low heat for a few minutes. Top pudding with almonds or stir them in. Cool in refrigerator.

Frozen Foods

Popsicles are proportioned just right for children and are the easiest "ice cream" of all to make. Since popsicles are so popular with children, they are a great way to establish new tastes.

Frozen yogurt and ice cream can be made at home for parties or just for the fun of it.

JUICE BARS

What could be simpler? Freeze any juice or combination of juices into popsicle molds.

FRUITY BARS

Mix any juice with chunks of fruit. Add honey if needed. Freeze in popsicle molds.

SEED BARS

Add ½ cup ground seeds to each cup of juice. For variety, add mashed banana to the mixture. Freeze in popsicle molds.

YOGURT SURPRISE

2 cups yogurt
½ cup concentrated orange juice
1 tsp. nutritional yeast
2 T. chopped walnuts
    Combine and freeze in popsicle molds.

CAROB POPS

1 cup milk
½ cup yogurt
1 egg
1 T. carob powder
1 T. nutritional yeast
2 T. ground seeds
1 T. lecithin (optional)

Combine and freeze in popsicle molds.

This recipe can be altered by adding 2 T. peanut butter
and/or ½ banana. Carob absorbs the taste of the yeast so it can
be added without fear of ruining the taste.

FROZEN YOGURT

2 cups yogurt
¼ cup honey
¾ cup pureed fruit

Use fresh fruit if possible, but, if unavailable, use frozen,
unsweetened fruit. Chill yogurt mixture for a few hours in the
refrigerator. Then proceed with the directions on an ice cream
machine.

Surprisingly, carob frozen yogurt is good. Just add carob
powder instead of fruit.

HONEY ICE CREAM

Substitute honey for sugar in any recipe, and decrease the
liquid just a bit. Be sure to use lots of fresh fruit puree (or more
of whatever flavoring you are using), because honey has a more
distinctive flavor than sugar. Try to decrease the amount of
honey used in ice cream recipes and increase the fruit (or
whatever) flavoring over a period of time, so that sweetening is
less concentrated.

Rolls, Muffins, and Quick Breads

I f you do not have time to bake, there are many excellent multi-grain breads on the market, although you will have to sacrifice some freshness. If you have a natural bakery in your town, buy your bread from them, rather than bread in a health food store that has been shipped in from another city. Some natural bakeries even grind their own flour and use it the same day! If you have such a bakery near you, stick with it.

Some rainy afternoon try making your own bread for fun. Once you have mastered the art of breadmaking, you will probably *make* time to bake it each week. There are endless variations to experiment with, and your family will keep bugging you to make homemade bread.

New World [brand name] has a fabulous multi-grain bread mix, full of many different nutritious flours. I use this whenever I make homemade bread because it is convenient and fool proof.

If you are truly adventurous, search out recipes and come up with your own creations. I recommend *The Complete Book of High Protein Baking*, by Martha Ellen Katz (Ballantine 1975).

There are so many excellent natural bread cookbooks available, that I am only including recipes for quick breads here.

Quick breads of high quality are almost impossible to find. Even if they were easy to find, they could not compare to those you can mix up yourself at home.

CORN BREAD

¾ cup corn meal
¼ cup protein powder
¼ cup wheat germ
2 tsp. baking powder
½ tsp. baking soda
½ tsp. sea salt

¾ cup yogurt
1 T. honey
2 T. melted butter
1 egg
½ cup shredded carrots

Mix dry ingredients and liquid ingredients separately. Combine the two just until they are mixed. Stir in shredded carrot, and pour into a buttered, square baking pan. Bake at 375° for about ½ hour.

CHEESE BISCUITS

1 cup whole wheat pastry flour
½ cup ground wheat germ
½ cup milk powder
2½ tsp. baking powder

½ tsp. sea salt
1 cup grated cheese
4 T. butter
¾ cup yogurt

Sift flour. Gently stir in the remaining dry ingredients. Mix in cheese. Cut butter into mixture using two knives or your fingertips. When the mixtue is crumbly, add yogurt. Knead dough for about ½ minute with a light touch. Then roll out about ½ inch thick, press with a biscuit cutter, and place on a buttered baking sheet. Bake at 400° for about 15 minutes.

BANANA NUT BREAD

⅓ cup butter
½ cup honey
2 beaten eggs
¼ cup milk powder
1 T. nutritional yeast
½ cup nut flour

4 mashed bananas
¼ cup wheat germ
¾ cup whole wheat pastry flour
2 tsp. baking powder
½ tsp. vanilla
½ cup chopped almonds

Preheat oven to 350°. Cream butter and honey. Add eggs and mashed banana. Combine dry ingredients and mix with banana mixture. Stir in vanilla and nuts. Bake in a 9 x 5 x 3-inch loaf pan for about an hour.

Buckwheat Pancakes

¼ cup Fearn Soy-O [brand name] buckwheat pancake mix
2 T. nutritional yeast
2 T. milk powder   1 egg
¼ cup wheat germ   1 T. melted butter
¼ cup seed flour   ¾ cup milk

Combine dry and liquid ingredients separately, then mix together with a few quick strokes. Cook as usual, using butter or margarine. Serve with lots of butter and real maple syrup.

Seed Pancakes

3 eggs
¾ cup seed or nut flour
Splash of milk

Beat eggs with a fork, then mix in seed flour, using more if needed for the right consistency. Cook as usual, but do not use oil; butter and margarine work better. Serve with lots of butter and real maple syrup. These pancakes are great for a fast meal — just keep seed flour on hand in your refrigerator. Add a pinch of cinnamon for a change of taste.

Apple-Carrot Muffins

¼ cup honey
1 egg
¾ cup milk
¼ cup safflower oil
1¼ cups whole wheat pastry flour
¾ cup seed flour
¼ cup wheat germ
½ cup milk powder
2½ tsp. baking powder
¼ cup shredded carrot
¼ cup shredded apple
½ tsp. cinnamon

Mix honey, egg, milk, and oil. Combine dry ingredients with honey mixture. Stir in shredded carrot and apple. Bake at 325° for about 20 minutes.

NUTTY MUFFINS

¼ cup butter
¼ cup honey
½ cup peanut butter
1 beaten egg
⅔ cup milk
½ cup seed flour
½ cup milk powder
2 T. nutritional yeast
½ cup whole wheat pastry flour
½ cup wheat germ
½ cup chopped nuts

Combine butter, honey, peanut butter, egg, and milk. Mix dry ingredients, then add to peanut butter mixture. Stir in peanuts. Butter muffin tins and fill ⅔ full. Bake at 325° for 20 minutes.

HONEY BRAN MUFFINS

3 T. safflower oil
¼ cup honey
1¼ cup milk
1 egg
1½ cups bran
¼ cup milk or protein powder
¼ cup wheat germ
¼ cup seed flour
¼ cup whole wheat pastry flour
2 T. nutritional yeast
2½ tsp. baking powder
½ cup raisins or chopped nuts (optional)

Combine liquid ingredients and combine with dry ingredients with a few quick strokes. Stir in nuts or raisins. Bake at 350° for about 20 minutes.

CINNAMON ROLLS

Don't become frightened at the prospect of making these delicious rolls. They are not difficult to make, just time consuming, because you must wait for them to rise. These are great for a rainy afternoon with bored children. You may wish to double the recipe so you can freeze some for a not-so-dreary day!

The Dough

3 T. warm water
2 T. bakers yeast
¼ cup melted butter
⅓ cup honey
2 eggs
1½ tsp. sea salt
2½ cups whole wheat flour (*not* pastry flour)
¼ cup seed flour
½ cup soy flour or protein powder
2 T. nutritional yeast
¼ cup wheat germ
1 cup warm water

Dissolve bakers yeast in 3 T. warm water and 1 tsp. honey for 5 minutes. Combine butter, honey, eggs, and sea salt with yeast mixture. Mix remaining dry ingredients, and add to honey mixture, alternating with warm water until it is well mixed. Knead dough on a floured board. Place dough in a bowl, brush top with melted butter, cover, and allow to rise in a warm place until double in bulk (about 90 minutes).

The Filling

½ cup melted butter
¾ cup honey
2 T. cinnamon
1 cup chopped walnuts
½ cup raisins

Roll out dough into a rectangular shape. Spread on filling and roll like a jelly roll. Cut dough into 2 inch wide pieces and place on an oiled baking sheet.

The Topping

¼ cup melted butter
2 T. honey
1 tsp. cinnamon

Brush topping onto cinnamon rolls. Allow them to rise once more in a warm place for ½ hour. Bake at 325° for about ½ hour.

Cakes and Pies

Cakes

Cakes made with whole wheat flour and honey are heavier than the white flour and sugar variety. Since it is even more difficult to get them to rise with concentrated ingredients, variety flours should be used in moderation so the cake will rise properly.

CARROT CAKE

½ cup butter
¾ cup honey
2 beaten eggs
½ cup yogurt
¾ cup whole wheat pastry flour
½ cup seed flour
¼ cup wheat germ
1 T. nutritional yeast
1 tsp. soda
1½ tsp. cinnamon
¾ cup shredded carrots
¼ cup crushed pineapple
½ cup chopped walnuts

Preheat oven to 325°. Cream butter and honey. Mix in eggs and add yogurt. Combine dry ingredients, then mix with honey mixture. Stir in carrots, pineapple, and nuts. Pour into buttered 9 x 13 inch pan, and bake at 325° for about an hour.

Pound Cake

1 cup butter
¾ cup honey
4 beaten eggs
2 T. lemon juice
2 T. grated lemon rind
¾ cup whole wheat pastry flour
¼ cup milk powder
¼ cup nut flour
¼ tsp. baking powder
pinch of sea salt

Cream butter thoroughly. Slowly add honey and beat well. Beat in eggs one at a time, then add lemon juice and rind. Mix dry ingredients, and slowly add to honey-butter mixture on a low speed. Line a buttered 9 x 5 x 3-inch loaf pan with waxed paper and bake at 300° for 1¼ hours.

Lemon Yellow Cake

⅓ cup butter
1 cup honey
2 eggs, separated
1 cup milk
2 T. lemon juice
2¾ cups whole wheat pastry flour
¼ cup nut flour
¼ cup milk powder
1 T. baking powder
½ tsp. salt
grated rinds of 2 lemons

Cream butter and honey. Add egg yolks, milk, and lemon juice. Combine dry ingredients, then add slowly to honey mixture. Add lemon rinds. Beat egg whites and fold into batter. Pour into two 8-inch layer cake pans, or a tube pan, and bake for 25 minutes at 350°.

CAROB FUDGE CAKE

½ cup butter
1¼ cups honey
2 beaten eggs
½ cup yogurt
1½ cups whole wheat pastry flour
½ cup seed flour
¼ cup wheat germ
1 T. nutritional yeast
3 T. milk or protein powder
½ cup carob powder
½ tsp. soda
½ tsp. sea salt
1 tsp. baking powder
1 tsp. vanilla

Preheat oven to 350°. Cream butter and honey. Beat eggs and yogurt in a separate bowl. Combine dry ingredients and add alternately with yogurt mixture to the honey mixture. Add vanilla. Pour into two buttered round cake pans and bake at 350° for about ½ hour. Cool, and frost with Carob-Nut Frosting*.

CAROB CUPCAKES

¼ cup butter
¾ cup honey
1 beaten egg
½ cup yogurt
½ cup carob powder
½ cup whole wheat pastry flour
½ cup seed flour
1 T. nutritional yeast
1 tsp. baking soda
½ tsp. vanilla
½ cup chopped almonds

Cream butter and honey, then beat in egg and yogurt. Mix dry ingredients and combine with honey mixture. Stir in vanilla and nuts. Fill cupcake papers in a muffin tin about ⅔ full. Bake at 350° for 15-20 minutes.

* Recipe in this chapter.

CAROB-COVERED ECLAIRS

This recipe is from *Cooking With Love and Wheat Germ*, by Jane Kinderlehrer (Rodale Press 1977).

1 cup boiling water
¼ lb. butter
1 cup brown rice flour (or any other flour you enjoy)
4 eggs

Preheat oven to 425°. Melt butter in boiling water, then stir in flour. Add eggs one at a time until the dough forms a ball in the center of the pan. Form dough into oblong shapes, and place on a buttered baking sheet in preheated oven for 5 minutes. Reduce heat to 325° and bake for ½ hour. Cool. Then fill with Lemon Pudding* or whipped cream. Top with Carob Syrup**.

GINGERBREAD

½ cup honey
½ cup butter
¾ cup molasses
3 beaten eggs
1 cup yogurt
¾ cup whole wheat pastry flour
½ cup soy flour or protein powder
¼ cup milk powder
1 cup seed flour
2 T. nutritional yeast
1 tsp. baking soda
2 tsp. cinnamon
1 tsp. ginger
1 tsp. allspice
½ cup chopped walnuts
½ cup raisins

Beat honey and butter. Add molasses, eggs, and yogurt. Combine dry ingredients and mix with molasses mixture. Add nuts and raisins. Pour into a buttered 9x13-inch baking pan.

* Recipe in this chapter.
** Recipe in Chapter Twelve.

Bake at 325° for about an hour. This gingerbread is concentrated, but very delicious. My husband and son devour the entire batch within a day or two!

CAROB BROWNIES

½ cup butter
½ cup honey
½ cup carob powder
2 egg yolks
¼ cup whole wheat pastry flour
¼ cup milk powder
½ cup seed flour
1 T. nutritional yeast
½ cup chopped nuts
1 tsp. vanilla
2 beaten egg whites

Melt butter and mix in carob powder and honey over low heat. Remove from saucepan and allow to cool slightly. Then add egg yolks gradually to carob mixture. Mix dry ingredients and combine with carob mixture. Add nuts and vanilla. Fold in egg whites. Pour into an 8-inch pan and bake at 350° for about 35 minutes.

Cake Frostings

Children love to poke their fingers into the icing and steal a taste. No reason to deprive them of this pleasure, but frostings need added milk powder to help balance out the large amounts of sweetening. Use seeds and nuts to help boost the nutritional value.

To decorate a cake with colored frosting, use the natural colorings described in Chapter Eight.

CREAM CHEESE FROSTING

Blend:
12 oz. cream cheese
4 oz. yogurt
2 T. milk powder
juice of ½ lemon
2 T. grated lemon rind
¼ cup honey

This light-colored frosting may be colored for decoration.

Carob-Nut Frosting

Blend:
½ cup butter
½ cup honey
½ cup milk powder
2 T. carob powder
¼ cup chopped almonds

Peanut Butter-Banana Frosting

Blend:
½ cup peanut butter
1 T. nutritional yeast
¼ cup butter
⅔ cup honey
½ cup milk
½ mashed banana

Banana-Coconut Frosting

Blend:
2 mashed bananas
1 tsp. lemon juice
2 T. butter
¼ cup coconut
¾ cup honey
½ tsp. vanilla

Orange Frosting

Blend:
½ cup yogurt
¼ cup honey
1 T. butter
2 T. concentrated frozen orange juice
½ cup milk powder

Butter Frosting

¾ cup butter
½ cup honey
½ cup milk powder
optional flavoring: vanilla, lemon, mint

Blend butter and honey until smooth. Add milk powder slowly until desired consistency is reached.

This frosting is easily colored with natural dyes — beet juice, carrot juice, berry juice, chlorophyll, etc.† Since the colors are so much fun to experiment with, you may wish to make extra frosting so that you will have plenty to use for decorating the cake.

Pie Crusts

Homemade pies are easy to make and can be of high nutritional value. Use ground seeds, wheat germ, coconut, and ground nuts as the base for crumb crusts. Natural graham crackers can be used occassionally for a crumb crust but add a bit of wheat germ to boost it nutritionally.

To prebake a pie crust, coat with egg white, and bake at 350° for 5 minutes.

Seed and Nut Crust

Combine:
1 cup ground sunflower seeds
½ cup ground almonds
1 T. honey
1 T. melted butter

Press into a pie pan and prebake.

Cinnamon-Wheat Germ Crust

Combine:
½ cup wheat germ
1 cup seed flour
1 T. honey
1 T. safflower oil
1 tsp. cinnamon

Press into pie pan and prebake.

---

† Earthgrown natural food coloring may also be used

COCONUT CRUST

Combine:
1 cup shredded coconut
½ cup seed flour
1 T. honey
1 T. melted butter

Press into a pie pan and prebake.

ROLLED CRUST

1 cup whole wheat pastry flour
¼ cup seed flour
¼ cup wheat germ
¼ tsp. sea salt
½ cup cold butter
about 4 T. cold water

Combine first four ingredients. Cut butter into flour mixture until it resembles large crumbs. Add cold water 1 T. at a time, mixing well before adding the next one. When dough will hold together enough to form a ball you have added enough water. Chill dough. Roll out dough between two pieces of waxed paper about ⅛ inch thick. If dough should crack, add more water. Remove top sheet of waxed paper and place pie pan upside down on top of dough. Flip over and crimp edges. Double recipe for a two-crust pie.

Pie Filling

Fillings for pies may be puddings, custards, fruits, or vegetables. Pies are fun to experiment with. Enjoy creating your own natural recipes with the flavoring your family likes best.

BERRY PIE FILLING

4 cups berries (fresh or frozen, unsweetened)
½ cup honey
4 T. arrowroot powder

Combine honey and arrowroot, heat gently on top of stove. Mix in berries then pour into pie shell. Dot with butter. Cover with crust and bake at 375° for 45 minutes.

APPLE CRISP

4-6 sliced, unpeeled apples	¼ cup wheat germ
2 T. lemon juice	¾ cup whole wheat pastry flour
1 tsp. arrowroot powder	1 tsp. cinnamon
¾ cup seed flour	¼ cup melted butter
½ cup rolled oats	¼ cup honey

Sauté apples in butter on top of the stove. Mix lemon juice with arrowroot. Stir into apple mixture, cooking a bit longer. Mix honey and butter, then stir into mixed dry ingredients. Place apple mixture in a buttered pan and top with crumbly oatmeal mixture. Bake at 350° for about 30 minutes. Serve warm with cheese, yogurt, honey ice cream, or whipped cream.

APPLE PIE FILLING

thinly sliced unpeeled apples (enough to fill crust)
½ cup honey

1 T. lemon juice	1 tsp. cinnamon
2 T. apple juice	2 tsp. arrowroot powder

Combine and cook mixture until it thickens. Then pour into a crumb crust. Top with natural graham cracker crumbs and dot with butter. Bake at 350° for about 45 minutes.

CAROB-BANANA PIE FILLING

Fill a crumb crust with Carob-Banana Pudding*. Serve with whipped cream.

PECAN PIE FILLING

⅓ cup butter	2 T. molasses
¾ cup real maple syrup	1½ cups pecan halves
3 beaten eggs	1 tsp. vanilla

Cream butter and maple syrup. Beat eggs into syrup mixture. Add remaining ingredients. Pour into a prebaked pie crust and bake for 30 minutes at 375°.

* Recipe in this chapter.

Pumpkin Pie Filling

2 cups pumpkin
2 T. melted butter
1½ cups cream
¾ cup milk powder
2 eggs
½ cup honey or real maple syrup
1½ tsp. pumpkin pie spice

Combine and pour into a prebaked pie shell. Bake at 425° for 15 minutes, then reduce heat to 325° for about 45 minutes.

Recipe Index

For convenience in locating recipes with asterisks, the following is a list of all recipes in this book by their special names.